# Impacts and Interventions

# Impacts and Interventions

## The HIV/AIDS Epidemic and the Children of South Africa

*Edited by*
*Jeff Gow and Chris Desmond*

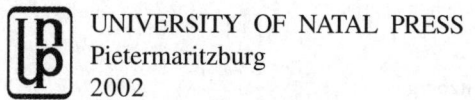
UNIVERSITY OF NATAL PRESS
Pietermaritzburg
2002

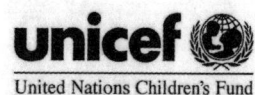
United Nations Children's Fund

Published by
University of Natal Press
Private Bag X01
Scottsville 3209
South Africa
Email: books@nu.ac.za
Website: www.unpress.co.za

© 2002 UNICEF

ISBN 1-86914-019-2

All rights reserved. No part of this publication may be reproduced or transmitted in any form or by any means, electronic or mechanical, including photocopying, recording or any information storage system, without prior permission in writing of the publishers.

The views expressed in this publication are those of the author(s) and not necessarily those of UNICEF.

Health Economics and HIV/AIDS Research Division (HEARD)
University of Natal, Durban, KwaZulu-Natal, South Africa
Director: Alan Whiteside
9th Floor
Shepstone Building
University of Natal
Durban 4041
South Africa
Tel: + 27 31 260 2592
Fax: + 27 31 260 2587
Website: http://www.und.ac.za/und/heard

Cover design: Sumayya Essack
Cover photograph: David Larson

Printed by Interpak Books, Pietermaritzburg

# Contents

| | |
|---|---|
| List of Contributors | vii |
| Acknowledgements | ix |
| Foreword *by Alan Whiteside* | xi |
| Foreword *by Giovanni Andrea Cornia and Jesper Morch* | xiii |
| List of Abbreviations | xv |

**Introduction**
| | | |
|---|---|---|
| Chapter 1 | Children and HIV/AIDS<br>*Jeff Gow, Chris Desmond and Deborah Ewing* | 3 |

**Part One  Impacts**
| | | |
|---|---|---|
| Chapter 2 | Epidemiological and Demographic<br>*Rob Dorrington and Leigh Johnson* | 13 |
| Chapter 3 | Health<br>*Sonja Giese* | 59 |
| Chapter 4 | Welfare<br>*Deborah Ewing* | 79 |
| Chapter 5 | Education<br>*Peter Badcock-Walters* | 95 |
| Chapter 6 | Households<br>*Jeff Gow and Chris Desmond* | 111 |

**Part Two  Interventions**
| | | |
|---|---|---|
| Chapter 7 | Mitigating the Impacts with a Focus on Government Responses<br>*Judith Streak* | 147 |
| Chapter 8 | Treatment of HIV/AIDS and Related Illnesses<br>*Neil McKerrow* | 175 |
| Chapter 9 | Preventing Transmission of HIV<br>*Rose Smart* | 189 |

**Conclusion**
| | | |
|---|---|---|
| Chapter 10 | Time for the Next Steps<br>*Jeff Gow and Chris Desmond* | 207 |

| | |
|---|---|
| Annex: AIDS, Public Policy and Child Well-being | 209 |

# Contributors

**Peter Badcock-Walters**
Research Associate, Health Economics and HIV/AIDS Research Division (HEARD), University of Natal, Durban, KwaZulu-Natal, South Africa.

**Chris Desmond**
Research Fellow, Health Economics and HIV/AIDS Research Division (HEARD), University of Natal, Durban, KwaZulu-Natal, South Africa.

**Rob Dorrington**
Director, Centre for Actuarial Research, University of Cape Town, Rondebosch, South Africa.

**Deborah Ewing**
Partner, Immediate Communication, Durban, KwaZulu-Natal, South Africa.

**Sonja Giese**
Researcher, The Child Health Policy Institute (CHPI), Department of Paediatrics and Child Health, University of Cape Town, Rondebosch, South Africa.

**Jeff Gow**
Research Associate, Health Economics and HIV/AIDS Research Division (HEARD), University of Natal, Durban, KwaZulu-Natal, South Africa and Lecturer, School of Economics, University of New England, Armidale, Australia.

**Leigh Johnson**
Researcher, Centre for Actuarial Research, University of Cape Town, Rondebosch, South Africa.

**Neil McKerrow**
Paediatrician, Greys Hospital, Pietermaritzburg, KwaZulu-Natal, South Africa.

**Rose Smart**
Research Associate, Health Economics and HIV/AIDS Research Division (HEARD), University of Natal, Durban, KwaZulu-Natal, South Africa.

**Judith Streak**
Chief, Children's Budget Project, The Institute for Democracy in South Africa (IDASA), Cape Town, South Africa.

# Acknowledgements

This book arose out of research work that was commissioned by UNICEF South Africa from the editors when both were working at HEARD. We organised and supervised the South African country case study of a global study looking at the long term impacts of HIV/AIDS on children and the policy response.

Many people have contributed to this book and we would like to acknowledge their input.

UNICEF Innocenti Research Centre, Florence, Italy – Giovanni Andrea Cornia had overall direction of the global study. Fabio Zagonari, University of Bologna also contributed, as did Mahesh Patel from the Nairobi office of UNICEF.

UNICEF South Africa – Gloria Kodzwa and Kiari Liman-Tinguiri were our initial contacts at UNICEF and strong supporters of our involvement in the study. Country Representative, Jesper Morch and Micaela Marques de Sousa were also supportive. Rina Gill was instrumental in helping to get the book published.

HEARD staff – Gavin George, Samantha Willan, Tim Quinlan, Madeline Freeman, Ace Ngcobo and Alan Whiteside all assisted in the gestation and production of the book.

The contributors – for their fulsome co-operation and worthy words. Shirin Motala provided important fieldwork assistance. Monica Holst and Anthea Dallimore – for their data collection efforts for the household impact chapter.

The Publisher, Glenn Cowley, and the staff of the University of Natal Press, especially Trish Comrie and Sally Hines.

Jeff Gow and Chris Desmond
June 2002

# Foreword

## Alan Whiteside

Currently there are an estimated 300 000 AIDS orphans in South Africa as a result of the HIV/AIDS epidemic. By 2015 there will be almost 2 million AIDS orphans, an increase of over 600 percent. This is clearly a catastrophe of considerable magnitude. These children, growing up without parental guidance, will for the most part be unloved, uncared for, unsocialised and uneducated. Extended families absorbing these children are finding themselves with fewer and fewer resources, psychological and financial, for existing family members.

And yet we have ample warning of what is going to happen. We know roughly how many infections there are, how many deaths there will be, when and where they will occur. We know that we are going to face this burden. One has to ask why is there the lack of planning and of response? Until very recently no one, from international agencies through to local departments of welfare in the national and provincial government, had begun to grapple with the magnitude of the problem, the resources required to respond to it, and the mechanisms with which to do this.

The Health Economics and HIV/AIDS Research Division (HEARD) has been deeply concerned about the orphan issue for a number of years. Early work by Desmond and Gow looked at the costs in providing different types of children's care. In 2000 we were invited to participate in a UNICEF project on 'Policies to sustain child welfare over the long term in countries affected by HIV/AIDS', which took place over 11 months. As part of this project we commissioned a number of papers and these were then sum-marised and presented in Florence in September 2001. Given that so much work had been done it seemed a pity to leave it as just a summary statement and we decided to approach both UNICEF and the organisers of the conference, to see if they would approve our editing these papers and putting them into book form. I am delighted to be able to write this brief foreword introducing the book which has been produced as a result of this collaboration. I should like to express my sincere thanks to Professor Giovanni Andrea Cornia for his permission to put together the papers in a book form, and to him and Jesper Morch for writing the short foreword that follows this section. I would also like to express my sincere appreciation to Rina Gill of UNICEF Pretoria for her support – this extended beyond the financial to the moral and administrative. Without her and the staff at UNICEF this project would have not been possible.

As Director of HEARD I would also like to express my gratitude to Jeff Gow and Chris Desmond for their hard work in putting this book together, and to the University of Natal Press for publishing it.

AIDS is without doubt the most important crisis facing this part of southern Africa. There are challenges around care, prevention and mitigation. Nowhere, though, is the challenge more important with regard to children and the next generation. South Africa has experienced one lost generation, we cannot afford another. This book goes a long way towards addressing these issues. I commend it to you and urge you to read it with the care and attention it deserves.

Director<br>
Health Economics and HIV/AIDS Research Division (HEARD)<br>
University of Natal, Durban<br>
South Africa

# Foreword

*Giovanni Andrea Cornia and Jesper Morch*

This book deals with one of the greatest and still unresolved challenges of our time, i.e. the damage caused by HIV/AIDS to the wellbeing and smooth functioning of the societies affected. With the rise in prevalence rates at antenatal clinics exceeding 40 per cent, as in areas of KwaZulu-Natal, and with a nation-wide adult prevalence rate in excess of the critical threshold of 20 per cent, South Africa is one of the countries most severely affected by this new challenge.

While the overall problem posed by AIDS has now been recognised, if belatedly, in most countries including South Africa, the specific impact of HIV/AIDS on children remains – with the exception of the orphans problem – poorly documented, analysed and understood. Indeed, most of the recent debate on the impact of HIV/AIDS has focused on adult prevalence and death rates, ways to control the spread of the disease over the short term, and its economic impact. This approach may have diverted our attention from the recent changes in infant mortality, enrolment rates and child malnutrition, from the new ways through which HIV/AIDS affects child wellbeing, and from the mitigating effects of old and new policy responses that need to be introduced under these circumstances. Indeed, the study of the impact of HIV/AIDS on infants and young children has been comparatively neglected in a period during which many indicators of child wellbeing have deteriorated sharply in close to half of the AIDS affected countries. In Botswana for instance, while under five mortality rates declined from 84 to 58 per thousand between 1980 and 1990 it rose to 101 by 2000, more than erasing in the latter decade the gains in child mortality recorded during the entire 1980s.

Even when the analysis has focused on children, it concentrated mainly on the children of families directly affected by HIV/AIDS. However, AIDS affects all children, whether from AIDS-affected families or not. The weakening of primary healthcare and educational services due to mounting death rates, disease prevalence and low morale among service providers is imposing large long-term costs on all children. The same can be said of their widespread impoverishment or the rise in school and healthcare fees imposed by governments suffering from fiscal crises, or of the rise in the price of essential drugs and other key items.

A third gap in the literature concerns the nature of the policies to mitigate the impact of HIV/AIDS on children. So far, the debate has been dominated by the prevention of HIV through information campaigns, the palliative care of infected adults and support to community-based responses for the care of orphans. Reliance on the communities is certainly rational but suffers from at least two problems. While reliance on community care is justified when few members of a community are affected, this becomes grossly insufficient when many are affected simultaneously. Broader insurance and redistributive policies, including income transfers from the central government, are needed.

Public policy ought therefore to play a more pro-active and longer-term role than it has done so far. There are several programmes and policies that would benefit children directly or indirectly that need to be given priority, including a strengthening of primary healthcare as the main vehicle for the treatment of all child diseases, both AIDS and non-AIDS related; a rapid expansion of prevention of mother-to-child-transmission programmes; a gradual expansion of the treatment of mothers and other adults with generic anti-retrovirals; the accelerated formation of teachers, doctors, technical staff, administrators and so on to prevent the medium-term collapse of public services and of the economy; the waiver of user fees in the social sector and stronger budgetary priorities in the allocation of domestic and international resource in favour of AIDS programmes. Government support to families with orphans, foster families, nutritional programmes, poor relief and so on, may also play a role.

To help focus the attention of policy makers, communities, practitioners and scholars on the specific impact of AIDS on children, UNICEF sponsored in 2000 a global study in this area comprising nine country cases studies (six in Africa and three in Asia) and five sectoral contributions. Due to the richness of the statistical information it provides, the high quality of its analysis and its comprehensiveness, that of South Africa is one of the best contributions to the UNICEF overall study. We trust its finding will help also the South African authorities, practitioners, NGOs and communities in their difficult fight against AIDS. As such, we strongly recommend it to all those interested in defeating this terrible scourge.

Professor of Economics, University of Florence
Co-ordinator of the Global UNICEF Study on the Impact of HIV/AIDS on Children,
UNICEF Representative to South Africa, Pretoria

# Abbreviations

| | |
|---|---|
| ACESS | Alliance for Children's Entitlement to Social Security |
| AIDS | acquired immune deficiency syndrome |
| ANC | African National Congress |
| ARV | anti-retroviral |
| ASSA | Actuarial Society of South Africa |
| ATICC | AIDS Training, Information and Counselling Centre |
| CBO | community-based organisations |
| CDG | care dependency grant |
| CINDI | Children in Distress |
| CMR | under-five mortality rate |
| CRC | Convention on the Rights of the Child |
| CSG | child support grant |
| DOTS | Directly Observed Treatment, Short-Course |
| FG | foster grant |
| GDP | Gross Domestic Product |
| HBC | home-based care |
| HCBCS | home- and community-based care and support programme |
| HIV | human immunodeficiency virus |
| HIVSP | HIV/AIDS/STD Strategic Plan for South Africa 2000–2005 |
| IDC | Interdepartmental Committee on AIDS |
| IFP | Inkatha Freedom Party |
| IMR | infant mortality rate |
| IP | National Integrated Plan for Children Infected and Affected by HIV/AIDS |
| IS | Integrated Strategy |
| MTCT | mother to child transmission |
| MTCTP | mother-to-child-transmission prevention |
| MTEF | Medium Term Expenditure Framework |

| | |
|---|---|
| NACOSA | National AIDS Convention of South Africa |
| NGO | non-governmental organisation |
| NIV | National Institute of Virology |
| NPA | National Program of Action for Children |
| OVC | orphans and vulnerable children |
| PMA | Pharmaceutical Manufacturers Association |
| PPT | Periodic Presumptive Treatment |
| SADHS | South African Demographic and Health Survey |
| SAIMR | South African Institute of Medical Research |
| SAYP | South African AIDS Youth Programme |
| STD | sexually transmitted disease |
| TAC | Treatment Action Campaign |
| TB | tuberculosis |
| UN | United Nations |
| UNAID | Joint United Nations Programme on HIV/AIDS |
| USAID | The United States Agency for International Development |
| UNICEF | United Nations Children's Fund |
| VCT | voluntary counselling and testing |
| WHO | World Health Organisation |

# INTRODUCTION

# CHAPTER 1

# Children and HIV/AIDS

*Jeff Gow, Chris Desmond and Deborah Ewing*

## Introduction

The HIV/AIDS epidemic is one of the greatest humanitarian and development challenges facing the global community. It is particularly acute in sub-Saharan Africa. At present about 45 million people world-wide have been infected with HIV (UNAIDS, 2001). Over 85 per cent of these people live in Africa. The HIV/AIDS epidemic in Africa has impacted in many ways. One of the most long-term impacts is the creation of an estimated 13 million orphans by 2000 which will rise to 24 million by 2010 and reach 40 million by 2020 (UNAIDS, 2001). In the absence of parents the care and support of these children will fall to extended families, civil society and governments in the various African countries.

The most recent estimate of the number of children in South Africa, from the 1999 October Household Survey, is 17 891 164 children under the age of 18. Census 1996 estimated that there were 16 333 349 children. Both estimates imply that about 40 per cent of the country's total population are children.

In this book the United Nations definition of the child is used: children up to the age of 18. Furthermore, the broad framework of children's rights set out in the United Nations Convention on the Rights of the Child (CRC) – Survival, Development, Protection and Participation – is used to examine the impacts of the HIV/AIDS epidemic upon them. Therefore, in looking at the impact of HIV/AIDS on children, consideration is given to deprivation of rights in any of those categories.

Since 1994, the South African government has committed itself to protecting child rights. This commitment is articulated in its ratification of the Convention on the Rights of the Child and Section 28 of the Constitution. Section 28 sets out the rights that all children are entitled to. The four pillars of rights these institutions promise to deliver follow the United Nations convention of survival, development, protection and participation rights. Since

1994 a programme, known as the 'National Programme of Action for Children' (NPA) has been in place to translate these promises into reality.

A commitment to citizen's participation in the governance of South Africa and in decision making which impacts upon them is enshrined as a constitutional obligation on the South African state through the Bill of Rights and has been reiterated in various policy documents concerned with child and family wellbeing. According to the United Nations Convention on the Rights of the Child, Article 12, children have the right to participate in decisions that affect them, and due weight should be given to their opinions, according to their age and maturity. This includes the right to participate in decisions that impact on their lives.

The geographic focus of the book is South Africa. However, the impacts of the epidemic upon children are being replayed in nearly all of the countries throughout sub-Saharan Africa. Those countries in Eastern and Central Africa, which first experienced the full wrath of the epidemic during the 1990s, have experienced similar and worse impacts than those described in this book. However, the feature distinguishing of South Africa from these other countries is the capacity of civil society and government to respond to the epidemic. South Africa has the resources, both human and financial, within its people and government, to address the impacts and implement programmes to mitigate and overcome the worst effects of the epidemic.

This book has children as its focus. All children will be affected by the HIV/AIDS epidemic which is now reaping its toll on South Africa and will continue to do so for the foreseeable future. However, some children will be more adversely affected than others – most obviously, those children who are born HIV-positive or soon after birth acquire the virus. Without access to anti-retroviral drugs these children will live short lives and die usually in pain. The healthy children of HIV-positive parents will be adversely affected during their parents' illnesses and usually be faced with severe consequences once one or both of their parents die. The children of those families which take in orphans, often in very resource constrained situations to start with, will be adversely affected as less resources are available for their care and development. Even those children from unaffected households will be affected as their playmates leave school, through destruction of their households following death, or lose their friends as abandoned children are forced to fend for themselves and move away from their homes and villages in search of resources to survive.

Children suffer physical, emotional and developmental setbacks as a result of the epidemic.

## Physical impacts

UNICEF's State of the World's Children 2000 highlights the reversal in child and infant mortality rates in sub-Saharan Africa (UNICEF, 2001a). The statistics for South Africa show the child mortality rate (CMR) down from 130 per 1 000 in 1960, to 81 per 1 000 in 1990. According to UNICEF, by 1998, this figure had gone back up to 83 per 1 000. This figure is disputed as not including the latest national health data, putting the CMR at 59. If the latter is accurate, the most recent projections are even more shocking: they show the CMR will rise to 100 in the next couple of years – and remain around there until 2009. The infant mortality rate (IMR) in South Africa is over 50 per 1 000 (this is up from 45 in 1998, having been brought down from 89 in 1960, and compares to Cuba's seven). There is considerable provincial variation, with the Eastern Cape, KwaZulu-Natal, Free State and Mpumalanga all having a CMR over the national average.

Core indicators such as infant and child mortality rates, immunisation, and nutritional status of children have worsened. The latest data, and the projections based thereon, show a direct correlation between HIV/AIDS and both child and adult mortality indicators. The impact is highly visible and measurable at community and household levels in both urban and rural areas, although it does not yet form part of the national picture of the epidemic. The national statistics on the cause of childhood deaths cite diarrhoea as the cause of 25 per cent of under-five deaths and acute respiratory infection as the cause of ten per cent of such deaths. While these are commonly AIDS-defining diseases, the deaths cannot be isolated as AIDS-related. The official categorisation of deaths such that preventable but fatal childhood illnesses are recorded as natural causes also obstructs analysis.

The rise in the IMR/CMR is directly due to HIV/AIDS, that is through mother to child transmission (MTCT), and illustrates the vicious circle of the link between AIDS and poverty. A woman living in poverty is more vulnerable to HIV infection, less likely to be able to negotiate safe sex and does not have access to mother-to-child-transmission prevention (MTCTP) treatment if she becomes pregnant. She will also not have access to anti-retroviral drugs and other treatment and will therefore become sick and die sooner than a woman who can afford treatment. The HIV-positive child and his/her siblings in the impoverished family will then be orphaned and plunge into deeper poverty. The HIV-positive child is then likely to die without treatment before the age of five, while the uninfected child is more likely to die of preventable and treatable childhood illnesses related to poverty.

### Emotional/Psychological impacts

The HIV/AIDS epidemic is contributing to psychological problems, especially among young children. The emotional wellbeing of children is threatened. This is evidenced by the increase in numbers of children coming onto the streets – not only in the major cities but also in small towns. The incidence of drug abuse has increased while the age at which children are being exposed is decreasing. In HIV/AIDS-affected families relevant factors include bereavement and psychological depression in the surviving parent/caregiver, which tends to incapacitate them in child rearing, and to impair their ability to work, obtain food, and provide adequate meals for their children. There are severe psychological health impacts for children of bereavement due to AIDS – and indirect impacts from being cared for by someone who is exhausted, distressed and desperately poor. The effects of bereavement on children and on the way that AIDS-related illness and death is being explained (or not) to children can be devastating. There are increasing numbers of child-headed households due to the death of parents from HIV/AIDS. However, there is a lack of empirical data on this phenomenon including how serious the problem is and what the prevailing circumstances are which predispose children to becoming part of child-headed households.

**Developmental impacts**
Prior to the emergence of HIV, large numbers of children and families already lived in poverty. The epidemic is worsening and deepening the poverty experienced by the poorest children and families. Empirical evidence was lacking as to the extent of the impacts. However, these impacts are discussed in this book. HIV/AIDS is contributing to increased vulnerability to poverty.

An area of concern is the issue of children as caregivers. The media has cited many examples of children taking physical care of their ill HIV/AIDS-infected parents or relatives. Some organisations have responded to this by providing training to such children on how to avoid getting infected and by providing them with appropriate resources such as gloves, etc. However, many child rights activists are of the view that this may appear to be accommodating the situation rather than addressing the problem of lack of alternate care. A fundamental issue to be addressed is the question of why children have to take on responsibilities, which are beyond their capacity and in fact may be harmful in some or other way to their development.

Increasing numbers of children are leaving school due to AIDS-related poverty, despite free education since 1994. Although caregivers can insist on the right to free education, pressure from principals of impoverished schools to pay school fees (48 per cent of schools still do not have electricity) on equally impoverished parents is considerable. Currently 1.6 million school-age children are out of school. Without treatment intervention to improve and prolong life of HIV-positive mothers, the number of maternal AIDS orphans is expected to rise from some 300 000 currently to around 3 million by 2011. Taking into account the number of orphans, the increased care/dependency ratio due to these deaths, the level of impoverishment due to loss of breadwinners and the burden of care for those dying, the impact on education – recognised as providing the best chance of escape from poverty – is probably incalculable. All over sub-Saharan Africa, hard-won gains in school enrolment – and the returns on investments countries have made to improve education – are being eroded (UNICEF, 2000b).

### Case Study

Neli is eight and lives in Msinga, the poorest district in KwaZulu-Natal. Her father was shot dead when she was a baby and her mother died of an AIDS-related illness in October 1999. Neli's grandfather was murdered several years ago. She lives with her aunt and her granny, who is now seriously ill – her hospital card shows she has been treated for tuberculosis and has lost ten kilos in weight in eight months.

Neli says: 'My mother was very sick before she died. Now my granny is ill. I have been very worried since my mom died. I don't understand why she died – my granny didn't say anything. I was very sad. I don't cry any more but I find it difficult to sleep alone.'

'We don't have enough to eat at home. We eat only mealie meal. Sometimes I get sick with stomach ache. I don't think anyone can really help us here.'

Neli says she has never been to school. 'My granny doesn't get pension yet. My uncle works in Johannesburg and sometimes he gives us money. My granny said she will send me to school when she gets her pension. That will help. I want to be able to read. I want to grow up, then I will go to work in Johannesburg as a nurse.'

## *Outline of the book*

The book is divided into two parts. Part One examines the impacts of the HIV/AIDS epidemic on the three main areas of child development which government has some direct influence upon: health, welfare and education. It closes with an examination of the impact of the epidemic within households in a small, rural community of KwaZulu-Natal.

Chapter Two involves a detailed analysis of past trends in HIV prevalence and current projections. It includes discussion on the underlying factors driving the epidemic and its geographical variation. Projections through to 2010 are generated using the ASSA2000 model, of both the prevalence and demographic impact at a national and provincial level. These projections are then compared to the different demographic and prevalence projections generated by alternative models. Finally, an estimate of the number of orphans is made.

Chapter Three gives a detailed examination of the impact of HIV on the health of children. It commences with a discussion of HIV transmission and progression and the link between HIV and the nutritional status of children. The chapter examines not only the provision of healthcare to the infected, but also the ability of the system to maintain other services as overall demand increases dramatically. The impact on orphan services is discussed in light of this growing demand.

Chapter Four presents a critical discussion of the impact of HIV/AIDS on child welfare, especially related to poverty. This is done by examining the impact on key indicators. This involves assessing the impact to date and discussion of expectations of future impacts of the epidemic on poverty levels. This includes reference to household level impacts on income and possible community level impacts.

Chapter Five is a detailed discussion of the impacts of HIV/AIDS on the education system. The focus is twofold: children as students and adults as educators. First, examination of the impacts of HIV within the family, especially the loss of resources for education and the implications for effective participa-tion by children in those circumstances. The second focus is on HIV as a management issue affecting the functioning of the infected educators and the sustainability of the system with large numbers of educators both ill and dying.

Chapter Six discusses the impacts of HIV/AIDS on three types of households: those with an orphan present, those with a seriously ill person present and control (those without either of the first two types of household). These households were located in the Bergville district of KwaZulu-Natal. This is the first published empirical evidence as to the impacts of the epidemic on households and in particular the impacts upon children in those households.

Part Two looks at the community and government interventions which have been undertaken to try to prevent the transmission of HIV, treat those infected and affected by HIV and look at what other actions have been undertaken to mitigate the impacts of the epidemic.

Chapter Seven involves a detailed analysis of government measures to mitigate the impact of HIV/AIDS, in particular upon children. The chapter attempts to trace the resource allocations of government to various programmes associated with mitigating impact. In the process it identifies a number of community and civil society responses.

Chapter Eight is a discussion of government and community interventions in the field of treatment of HIV/AIDS and related illnesses. This involves the outlining of official policies and observed realities or outcomes. The chapter also includes discussion on the treatment of tuberculosis (TB), sexually transmitted diseases (STDs) and access to anti-retroviral drugs.

Chapter Nine examines and critically discusses past and present interventions aimed at preventing the transmission and spread of HIV. The chapter focuses on government efforts in the area of prevention.

## References

Constitution of the Republic of South Africa Act 1996.
Statistics South Africa. 1998. 'The People of South Africa Population Census 1996'. Pretoria: Statistics South Africa.
Statistics South Africa. 2000. 'October Household Survey 1999'. Statistical Release PO317. Online. (accessed February 2002). http://www.statssa.gov.za/Statistical_Releases/Statistical_Releases.htm
United Nations. Undated. *Convention on the Rights of the Child.* New York: United Nations.
UNAIDS. 2001. *Report on the Global HIV/AIDS Epidemic.* Geneva: UNAIDS.
UNICEF. 2001a. *The State of the World's Children 2001.* New York: UNICEF.
UNICEF. 2001b. *The Progress of Nations 2000.* New York: UNICEF.
Whiteside, A. and C. Sunter. 2000. *AIDS: The Challenge for South Africa.* Cape Town: Human & Rousseau and Tafelberg.
World Bank. 1999. *Confronting AIDS: Public Priorities in a Global Epidemic.* New York: Oxford University Press.

# PART ONE

# Impacts

CHAPTER 2

# Epidemiological and Demographic

*Rob Dorrington and Leigh Johnson*

## Introduction

South Africa has one of the highest levels of HIV prevalence in the world and, with an estimated 4.2 million infections in 1999, is estimated by UNAIDS to have more HIV-positive citizens than any other country (UNAIDS, 2000). According to the Department of Health (2001) the figure for 2000 is 4.7 million, but for various reasons this is probably an underestimate. According to the ASSA2000 model the figure is closer to 5.3 million. Despite the South African epidemic having had a late start relative to the epidemic in other African countries, the epidemic has already reached catastrophic proportions in many parts of the country, and it is expected that prevalence levels will continue to rise for some years to come. Even so, there is still very little understanding of how best to manage the epidemic, or indeed, a comprehensive system of measuring the impact of the epidemic.

This chapter begins with a short description of the social epidemiology of the epidemic in South Africa. For more detail the reader is referred to *HIV Risk Factors: A Review of the Demographic, Socio-economic, Biomedical and Behavioural Determinants of HIV Prevalence in South Africa* by L. Johnson and D. Budlender (2002). This is followed by a description of the nature and reliability of the surveillance system in the country and an analysis of the spread of the epidemic to date. Based on these data the ASSA2000 model is used to project the population to 2010 and the results of this projection are compared, with those of three other models. The chapter concludes by briefly outlining the impact of the epidemic on the number of orphans.

## Social epidemiology of HIV/AIDS in South Africa

The first AIDS case in South Africa was diagnosed in 1982 (Department of

National Health and Population Development, 1994b) and since then the prevalence recorded by the national antenatal seroprevalence survey has risen steeply from less than one per cent in 1990 to nearly 25 per cent, ten years later. That the epidemic has spread so rapidly and so extensively in South Africa in particular is not surprising. Zwi and Cabral (1991) identified what they termed a high risk situation as one characterised by 'impoverishment and disenfranchisement, rapid urbanisation, the anonymity of urban life, labour migration, widespread population movements and displacements, social disruption, wars, especially counter-insurgency wars' (Marks, 2001). As Marks (2001) and Dorrington (1999) point out, on any scale of high-risk situations South Africa in the 1980s ranked near the top. A number of the factors that have contributed to the explosive rise in prevalence are explored below.

**Bio-medical factors**
The most significant bio-medical factor driving the epidemic is the high prevalence of sexually transmitted diseases (STDs). Genital sores and ulcers caused by these STDs greatly increase the risk of HIV transmission, and there is thus a significant correlation between levels of STD and HIV prevalence. The following figures bear testimony to the high levels of sexually transmitted infection:

- It is estimated that there were between 5 000 and 15 000 cases per 100 000 of syphilis in 1996. This compares with a rate of about 15 per 100 000 in the United States of America and the United Kingdom (Pham-Kanter et al., 1996).
- A study conducted in Carletonville found that 14 per cent of men, 22 per cent of women and 11 per cent of migrant mine workers were infected with syphilis, gonorrhoea or chlamydia (Williams et al., 2000a).
- Wilkinson et al. (1999a) estimate that 25 per cent of women in rural KwaZulu-Natal have at least one STD.
- According to the South African Demographic and Health Survey (SADHS) (Department of Health, 1999b) about 12 per cent of men reported having suffered from an STD in the last three months.

Levels of STD treatment are low for a number of reasons. Firstly, many STDs (particularly those affecting women) are asymptomatic, and even when symptoms occur, they may not be recognised as being due to infection. A study of pregnant women in KwaZulu-Natal, for example, found that although more than 50 per cent had at least one infection of the reproductive tract, none volunteered symptoms of an STD (Sturm et al., 1998). A second problem is that even when symptoms occur, individuals will often not seek treatment, either because treatment is inaccessible or because the infection is not regarded as being serious. To aggravate the situation further, treatment is often ineffective. Colvin et al. (1997) found, for example, that 90 per cent of workplace clinics in KwaZulu-Natal gave unsuitable or partial treatment for STDs. The high level of STD prevalence in South Africa and the rest of Africa is thus a consequence of poor education on symptoms and causes of STDs, poor access to treatment, and poor quality of treatment (Colvin, 2000).

The relationship between HIV prevalence and STD prevalence is demonstrated in Figure 2.1. HIV prevalence levels among pregnant women, estimated from the 1998 antenatal clinic survey (Department of Health, 1999a), are compared with percentages of men reporting having had painful urination, penile discharge or genital sores in the last three months from the South African Demographic and Health Survey (SADHS) (Department of Health, 1999b), in each of the nine provinces. With the exception of Gauteng and the Northwest, there is a pattern of high HIV prevalence in provinces with high STD prevalence, and lower HIV prevalence in provinces with low STD prevalence. The anomalous situation in Gauteng can probably be explained by the high degree of urbanisation and relatively universal access to healthcare; that in Northwest is a little more difficult to understand.

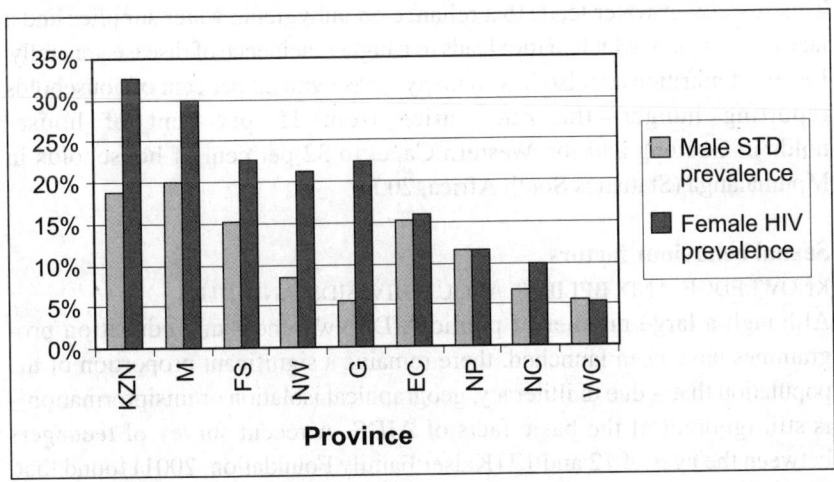

Source: Department of Health (1999a and 1999b)

Note: The abbreviations used here and in subsequent diagrams, for the nine provinces are as follows: KZN (KwaZulu-Natal), M (Mpumalanga), FS (Free State), NW (Northwest), G (Gauteng), EC (Eastern Cape), NP (Northern Province), NC (Northern Cape), WC (Western Cape).

**Figure 2.1 Comparison of STD and HIV prevalence levels (1998).**

It has been suggested that male circumcision may also be a significant bio-medical determinant of HIV incidence, the foreskin of the penis providing a vulnerable portal of entry for the virus. Evidence from elsewhere in Africa suggests that male circumcision tends to be associated with lower prevalence levels (Moses et al., 1990), and similar findings have been made in South Africa. In an urban study, Williams et al. (2000a) found that circumcision levels were highest among the Xhosa (53 per cent) and the Sotho (40 per cent), while levels were low among the Tswana (11 per cent) and the Zulu (12 per cent). They also found, when age differences were adjusted for, that HIV prevalence was significantly lower among circumcised men than among uncircumcised men ($p = 0.054$). This may explain the high prevalence of HIV in KwaZulu-Natal (inhabited mostly by Zulus) relative to that in the Eastern Cape (inhabited mostly by Xhosas), and may to some extent also explain the high prevalence in the urbanised black population, in which the practice of circumcision is becoming less common.

Sanitation and nutrition – to the extent that they influence the state of the immune system – may also affect the rate of transmission. Sanitation is a particular problem, with 65 per cent of the country receiving less than 500 mm of rainfall per year (500 mm being 60 per cent of the world average). In rural areas, 17 per cent of households have to fetch water from more than a kilometre away (Department of Welfare and Population Development, 1998). This scarcity of water leads to a reliance on unhygienic water supplies and a lack of sanitation, which in turn leads to a higher incidence of disease generally. Levels of nutrition are also low in many areas, with 22 per cent of households reporting hunger – the rate varies from 15 per cent of households in Gauteng and the Western Cape, to 32 per cent of households in Mpumalanga (Statistics South Africa, 2000).

**Sexual behaviour factors**
KNOWLEDGE AND BELIEFS ABOUT HIV/AIDS AND STDS
Although a large number of public AIDS awareness and education programmes have been launched, there remains a significant proportion of the population that – due to illiteracy, geographical isolation or misinformation – is still ignorant of the basic facts of AIDS. A recent survey of teenagers between the ages of 12 and 17 (Kaiser Family Foundation, 2001) found that:

- Levels of awareness of HIV/AIDS were high (91 per cent of respondents), but tended to be low in rural areas (86 per cent). The SADHS (Department of Health, 1999b) showed that among women between the ages of 15 and 49, 97 per cent had heard of AIDS, and of those who had heard of AIDS, 87 per cent knew that using condoms was a means of avoiding the disease

(the rate was again significantly different in urban and rural areas, at 91 per cent and 81 per cent respectively).
- Seven per cent of respondents said they believed that one could be cured of AIDS by having sex with a virgin, and 12 per cent believed that one could get HIV/AIDS from condoms.
- Thirteen per cent said they believed that traditional African medicine had a cure for AIDS, while 15 per cent believed that Western medicine had a cure.

Of equal concern is the more general ignorance regarding STDs. A study conducted by Williams et al. (2000a) found that among men and women with STDs, only 48 per cent of men and 37 per cent of women were aware that their STD could be passed on to their sexual partner.

SEXUAL ABUSE AND THE STATUS OF WOMEN
Since the new political dispensation in 1994, much political emphasis has been placed on the rights of women, and the need for gender equality. However, South Africa remains a fairly patriarchal society, in which women are vulnerable to sexual abuse. In 1998, South Africa had the highest per capita rate of reported rape in the world (115.6 for every 100 000 of the population), and on the common but highly debatable assumption that only one in every twenty rape cases are reported – close to one million acts of rape occur in South Africa every year (Rape Crisis Cape Town, 2001). Marital rape is particularly under-reported, with many relationships being characterised by violence and sexual abuse. Vundule et al. (2001) found, in a study of black teenagers attending antenatal clinics in Cape Town, that 72 per cent of girls reported having been forced to have sex at some stage, and 11 per cent reported having been raped. The South African National Youth Survey (Kaiser Family Foundation, 2001) also found that 39 per cent of sexually experienced girls had been forced to have sex, and 33 per cent reported being afraid of saying no to sex. In many cases, therefore, women have limited control over their sexual activity, and are thus more vulnerable to HIV infection.

PROSTITUTION AND HIGH-RISK FORMS OF SEXUAL BEHAVIOUR
Commercial sex workers are particularly at risk of infection. The first reason for this is the high number of sexual partners that they have (Rees et al. (2000) estimate that the average sex worker has 25 clients a week). The other reason is that sex workers are frequently forced to engage in high-risk forms of sexual intercourse, such as anal sex and dry sex.

Women practising dry sex use drying agents (including cloth, soap, detergents and traditional medicines) to tighten or dry their vaginas, in order to enhance the sexual experience of their male partners. It is believed that use of these agents increases a woman's chance of infection, and Williams et al. (2000a) found the HIV prevalence among women practising dry sex to be higher than that for women not practising it, both among sex workers (91 per cent against 66 per cent) and among non-sex workers (50 per cent against 41 per cent). Only 3.2 per cent of those women sampled were using drying agents, however, which suggests that the practice may not be as widespread as sometimes thought. Anal intercourse also greatly increases the risk of transmission, both for the penetrating partner and the receptive partner, and seven per cent of sex workers report practising anal sex at least once a week (Rees et al., 2000). Risk of transmission is further increased by lack of condom usage. Nineteen per cent of the sex workers sampled by Rees et al. reported using a condom less than 50 per cent of the time, 51 per cent reported using one between 50 and 75 per cent of the time, and only 30 per cent reported using one more than 75 per cent of the time.

It should be recognised that many women sell sex without regarding themselves as prostitutes, relying on regular financial support in return for sexual favours (Heywood, 1998). Other forms of sexual bartering are common. The South African National Youth Survey (Kaiser Family Foundation, 2001) found, for example, that 16 per cent of sexually experienced girls indicated having had sex for money, drink, food or gifts, and 20 per cent of sexually experienced boys reported having given a girlfriend pocket money, food or drink in exchange for sex. This widespread dependence on sex as a source of income creates an environment conducive to the rapid spread of HIV.

**Social risk factors**
MIGRATION PATTERNS
South Africa has experienced high levels of political and economic migration in recent decades, both between its provinces, and between itself and its neighbouring countries. Migration increases the extent of sexual networking, and thus facilitates the swift spread of the HIV/AIDS epidemic. This is demonstrated in a study of a rural community in KwaZulu-Natal: people who had recently changed place of residence were three times more likely to be HIV-positive than those who had not (Abdool Karim et al., 1992). It is therefore a concern that rates of migrant employment are as high as 60 per cent of males and a third of females, between the ages of 19 and 49, in some rural areas (Lurie et al., 1997).

One of the reasons for the high levels of migration is the forced removals initiated by the apartheid government. In the decade between 1975 and 1985 alone, more than 3.5 million black people were relocated to the twelve homelands (Platzky and Walker, 1985). Black people were prevented from settling permanently in the urban white areas and had to retain a rural base in these homelands. The poor agricultural and employment prospects in these areas forced many to seek work outside of the homelands on a migrant labour basis. Thus was created a substantial system of migrant labour. Zwi and Bachmayer (1990) estimated that in 1990 more than 2.5 million migrants, drawn from rural areas and neighbouring countries, were working in mines, factories and farms.

The mining industry in particular has been associated with high levels of migrant labour. In 1989 roughly 40 per cent of the workforce of the Chamber of Mines consisted of migrant workers from outside of South Africa (Ijsselmuiden et al., 1990). Crush (1995) reports that 90 per cent of all black employees in the gold mining industry are migrants, and that 89 per cent of these miners are accommodated in single sex hostels. Having to live separately from their spouses and regular sexual partners (many of whom reside in rural areas), those living in single sex hostels often engage in high-risk sexual activity with commercial sex workers.

Migrant workers who become infected in urban areas then pass the virus on to their partners when they return to the rural areas. Evidence suggests that transmission in the opposite direction may also occur: Lurie et al. (2000) have found that for nearly 40 per cent of discordant migrant couples, it is the female partner who is infected with HIV, not the male. This may indicate that women are forced to rely on sex to supplement their incomes while their partners are away for long periods.

POLITICAL TURMOIL AND WAR

Armed conflict has the effect of both displacing those seeking to avoid conflict, and destabilising the traditional power structures and value systems of the society. It also creates movements of armed forces between regions. Many of the armed forces of the apartheid government operated to the north of South Africa's borders, in Namibia and Angola. Many of the former revolutionary cadres also fought in these regions, and were incorporated into the national defence force and placed in bases all over the country after 1994 without any HIV testing. The return of these security forces, from areas of high HIV prevalence to military bases throughout the country, has no doubt contributed to the rapid growth of the epidemic in South Africa (Shell, 2000).

Within South Africa, KwaZulu-Natal has been particularly afflicted by violence and political conflict between ANC and IFP supporters. This violence has led to a collapse of social cohesion and a disintegration of parental authority (Humbridge, 1990), and is a significant factor contributing to the high levels of HIV prevalence in the province.

## OVERCROWDING AND POVERTY

Overcrowding and poverty are responsible for many of the social pressures that lead to high-risk sexual behaviour. The forced removals described previously led to an overcrowding in the former homelands, with resulting overgrazing, erosion and poor living conditions (Department of Health and Population Development, 1998). With the scrapping of the influx control laws (which prevented blacks from settling permanently in the urban white areas), there has been a steady trend towards urbanisation in the black population. The majority of these migrants have settled in large informal settlements on the peripheries of major cities.

Data from the 1999 October Household Survey, shown in Table 2.1, indicate that although access to basic services is improving, unemployment levels have risen in recent years (the official and expanded unemployment rates differ in that the former include only those who have been engaged in job seeking in the four weeks prior to the survey). Unemployment rates are particularly high in the black population, in rural areas, and among women, as Table 2.2 shows. These inequalities are a major force driving the epidemic.

**Table 2.1  Poverty indicators in 1996 and 1999.**

| Poverty indicators | 1996 | 1999 |
|---|---|---|
| % of households with access to piped water | 82.2 | 87.1 |
| % of households with access to sanitation | 87.1 | 85.8 |
| Literacy rate for 15–24 year olds | 94.9 | 95.8 |
| Official unemployment rate | 19.3 | 23.3 |
| Expanded unemployment rate | 33.0 | 36.2 |

Source: Statistics South Africa (2000)

**Table 2.2  Official unemployment rates, by race, gender and urban/rural status.**

| | Official unemployment rates (1999) | | | | | | |
|---|---|---|---|---|---|---|---|
| | Urban | | Rural | | Total | | |
| | Male | Female | Male | Female | Male | Female | Total |
| Asian | 14.6 | 16.4 | | | 14.5 | 17.2 | 15.6 |
| Black | 24.1 | 35.0 | 25.2 | 34.9 | 24.5 | 35.0 | 29.2 |
| Coloured | 15.7 | 19.1 | | | 13.4 | 17.5 | 15.2 |
| White | 4.4 | 5.3 | | | 4.4 | 5.1 | 4.7 |
| All | 18.4 | 25.8 | 22.7 | 32.3 | 19.8 | 27.8 | 23.3 |

Source: Statistics South Africa (2000)

**Economic factors**

Income is one of the most significant factors correlated with HIV prevalence. The relatively poor members of society are most affected by the epidemic, as most of the risk factors described above are linked to low socio-economic status. Heywood (1998) observes that the poor tend to work in high-risk occupations, and tend to be exposed to greater dangers in the course of their everyday life than the relatively wealthy. To many the threat of AIDS may seem remote relative to the stresses of their day-to-day lives. Being relatively uneducated, they are also less likely to know what AIDS is and how the virus is transmitted. Many do not have access to proper treatment for STDs, or cannot afford treatment. Of HIV/AIDS admissions to Somerset and Groote Schuur Hospitals between 1988 and 1993, only 48 per cent of heterosexual males had ever been employed, and of those who had been employed, 74 per cent had been employed in unskilled or semi-skilled labour (Maartens et al., 1997).

However, it should not be assumed that HIV/AIDS is a disease affecting exclusively the poor. It can be argued that as individuals earn more and their socio-economic status rises, they are able to attract greater numbers of sexual partners, which places them at greater risk of infection (Kinghorn and Steinberg, 1998). A study conducted in KwaZulu-Natal (albeit a small sample from two large towns) suggested that the prevalence level among pregnant women attending obstetricians in the private sector was not dissimilar from those of women attending public antenatal clinics, when race was controlled for (Wilkinson, 1999). The relatively low level of prevalence in the Northern Province, a very poor and rural region, suggests that the poorest of the poor – particularly the rural poor – are less affected than those with slightly higher levels of income. The relationship between HIV prevalence and income is therefore not a simple one.

Other figures released by companies suggest that even in the formal sector prevalence levels are high:

| | | |
|---|---|---|
| Gencor (mining) | 20% | (Heywood, 1996) |
| Impala Platinum Mine | 17% | (Whiteside and Sunter, 2000) |
| Illovo Sugar's Umfolozi Mill | 26% | (Caelers, 1999) |
| Transvaal Sugar Limited | 54% | (Caelers, 1999) |

The mining and agricultural sectors will clearly be hard hit, as might be expected, given the large numbers of migrant workers employed in these industries. One might similarly expect the defence force and transport industries to be particularly affected, as employment in these sectors is likely to be associated with long separations from family. However, the absence of these factors by no means ensures that a sector will not be hit hard. It is widely assumed, for example, that the teaching and nursing professions will be quite severely hit by the epidemic.

## The response of government

The history of the management of the AIDS epidemic is a sad one, and one that to some extent explains the high level of prevalence in the country. When the first AIDS cases were recorded in the early eighties among homosexual men, the government of the time disowned the problem on the grounds that it was illegal for men to be having sex with men. When the first cases occurred among the black heterosexual population, the government regarded it as a problem that the homelands, rather than they should be dealing with. The early stages of the epidemic were mismanaged by the previous government, and there is even evidence to suggest that senior members of the former defence force may have attempted to spread the epidemic in the black population (Shell, 2000). When the first democratically elected government came to power in 1994, its primary concern was to ensure transformation, and AIDS was only one item on a long list of challenges.

In the last decade government has been involved in a number of scandals and controversies over its handling of the AIDS crisis. The Sarafina II scandal of 1995 erupted when it was found that there were irregularities in the awarding of a tender for a musical stage production that was intended to tour the country with a message about AIDS, and that the production was of questionable value in terms of AIDS awareness. Soon afterwards, government supported research into Virodene – a treatment containing an industrial solvent known to cause liver damage. Moves to make AIDS a notifiable disease also generated much controversy. Most controversial of all, however, has been President Mbeki's questioning of the widely held view that HIV causes AIDS, and the establishment of a panel of experts – both mainstream and dissident – to explore this issue. More recently, government has come under attack for its reluctance to provide short-course anti-retroviral treatment to HIV-positive pregnant women. There has thus developed a perception that government is doing nothing about the epidemic (Whiteside and Sunter, 2000).

However, government's performance cannot be judged solely on the basis of media reports. Whiteside and Sunter (2000) identify the following as examples of the success stories:

- National STD management protocols have been adopted.
- Access to male condoms has improved significantly, with 150 million condoms being distributed free of charge in 1999.
- Thousands of secondary school teachers have been trained in HIV/AIDS.

- An annual HIV surveillance system was introduced in 1990, and has been used to derive national and provincial estimates of prevalence ever since. However, the government has shown a remarkable reluctance to allow independent researchers access to this data or to explain in detail the methods used to derive the national and provincial figures.
- In 1995 the AIDS Directorate was set up in the Department of Health. It obtained extensive funding from government and outside donors, and has embarked on a 'Beyond Awareness' campaign aimed at changing people's perceptions about not being at risk.

It is to be hoped that these positive measures will be sustained, and that they will reverse the effects of the mismanagement that characterised the early years of the epidemic.

## *Nature and reliability of the surveillance system*

Antenatal surveys are part of an initiative started by the World Health Organisation (WHO) and later taken up by UNAIDS for estimating the prevalence of HIV in the population. The national antenatal survey was first conducted in 1990 (Department of National Health and Population Development, 1995). It is recognised as being one of the most reliable surveys conducted by middle and low-income countries and certainly the best in sub-Saharan Africa, the epicentre of the epidemic.

The survey is an anonymous, voluntary (in that women are allowed to refuse to be tested), unlinked, cross-sectional survey of residual blood specimens which are collected for routine syphilis and rhesus testing, conducted among pregnant women attending public antenatal clinics for the first time during their current pregnancy. The survey is conducted concurrently over nine provinces during October each year. All provinces are said to 'follow the protocol closely' (Department of Health, 2001) although rumours still persist about some provinces either using a convenience sample (KwaZulu-Natal (Medical Research Council, 1998)), or sampling from all sites (Mpumulanga (Potgieter, 2000)).

The survey is based on a large scientifically selected sample of sentinel sites chosen to represent each province (currently over 16 000 specimens from 400 clinics are tested per year). The methodology was substantially revised in 1995 with the assistance of the Medical Research Council. In particular, improvements were made to the methodology of sampling, the quality control and the field procedures, phased in over a period from 1997 to 2000, to ensure that 'expected prevalence trends are not disrupted' (Department of Health, 2001).

The greatest weakness of the early antenatal surveys was the lack of a consistent sampling frame. Because blood was collected from laboratories there was no control over which clinics submitted samples nor over how patients were sampled. In addition, provinces used different sampling methodologies. These problems are graphically illustrated by the 1996 result for the North West – a three-fold increase for which there was no explanation. Efforts to calibrate, for the first time, the ASSA2000 AIDS and Demographic model to the deaths recorded by the Department of Home Affairs suggest that the antenatal clinic survey results in the early 1990s were biased upward, probably because of a concentration in the urban areas. This bias appears to have dissipated over the last ten years both as the sampling frame has improved and as the difference between the rural and urban prevalences narrowed.

The Department has yet to describe how the national estimate is derived from the provincial estimates. Elementary calculations show that they must have made a mistake with the weightings (at least) used in 1998 with the result that this figure was overstated by some two per cent. As much of the Department's assertion that the epidemic appears to have plateaued and to be under control is based on the pattern over the years 1998 to 2000, this error is leading to a misinterpretation of the epidemic and hence potentially undermining the effectiveness of intervention strategies.

In addition to this, a number of the provincial estimates from time to time look extremely out of line with the trend in the rest of the rates (for example Mpumalanga in 1998, Free State in 1999 and Gauteng in 2000) but the Department fails to make available sufficient detail of the survey (such as the number of specimens from the various health districts in each of the provinces over time) to enable independent checking of these anomalous results.

Currently the survey collects information on age, population group, level of education, parity of the woman providing the specimen and apparently (personal communication with Dr Lindiwe Makubalo, Chief Director in the Department of Health) in the most recent survey, the proportion of refusals. However, the Department of Health currently only makes public the overall results by province and the overall results by age. For the first time since the 1996 survey (Department of Health and Population Development, 1997) the department published their calculations (Department of Health, 2001) of the number of people estimated to be infected with the virus (4.7 million). Although it is not clear where they got the estimates of the mid-year population from it is clear, from these estimates and the assumptions used, that their estimate is on the low side.

According to the SADHS over 80 per cent of all pregnant women attend public antenatal clinics and over 85 per cent of these are black African women. In other words the survey under-represents women of other races, and since those women who do not attend public antenatal clinics attend private antenatal clinics the seroprevalence survey also under-represents richer women.

No STDs are notifiable, although congenital syphilis has been notifiable since 1991 and all government health facilities are obliged to routinely provide to the provincial informatics office a count of STDs treated. However, for various reasons these data tend to be poorly reported (Medical Research Council, 1998).

The only surveillance activity that is currently organised on a national basis is the annual HIV and syphilis seroprevalence survey. Syphilis serological tests have only been carried out since 1997. All other surveillance activity is provincially based. The national syphilis seroprevalence survey shows that at five per cent the prevalence has more than halved since 1997.

The Department is working on a number of other initiatives for monitoring the epidemic, namely, investigating the prevalence at private antenatal clinics, various behavioural surveillance activities, measuring HIV incidence rates, and introducing 'an expanded national surveillance system for STDs/HIV/AIDS'.

The South African Institute of Medical Research (SAIMR) in conjunction with the provincial health authorities has set up a system to measure STD syndromes in selected public health clinics. One major drawback is that it doesn't monitor private clinics and it is understood that many people prefer to use private doctors for the treatment of STDs.

The National Institute of Virology (NIV) compiles monthly reports of data submitted by seven diagnostic laboratories in the country. These reports give the number of positive tests for a variety of viruses including cytomegalovirus, herpes simplex virus and varicella zoster virus. However, these data are of limited usefulness since neither the total number of tests nor the criteria for doing the tests is given, although these data can indicate trends.

The largest group of people tested for HIV are the voluntary unpaid blood donors (approximately a million a year). Although figures on HIV and STD prevalence are published (by at least race and gender) they are very difficult to interpret owing to significant unknown biases (not least of which is the need for the South African Blood Transfusion Service to actively try to improve selection criteria to avoid donations by infected people). However, the trends in the data seem to mirror those in the antenatal data.

Although there have been several efforts to introduce local voluntary testing and AIDS reporting, the extent of under-reporting and variability of reporting to the voluntary AIDS reporting system results in the data being virtually useless.

## *Analysis of the spread of HIV and the demographic variations to date*

The HIV/AIDS epidemic spread into South Africa from two foreign sources. Initially the epidemic spread into the (mostly white) homosexual and bisexual population through contact with homosexuals in Western countries, the first homosexual AIDS cases in South Africa being recorded in 1982 (Sher, 1989). Schoub et al. (1988) report the first case of AIDS in the heterosexual population occurring in 1988. The epidemic is believed to have spread into the heterosexual population from central and southern African countries, through migrant workers, truck drivers and immigrants. The heterosexual and homosexual epidemics have remained largely independent, and are distinguished by distinct viral sub-types – sub-type B, common in Europe and the US, has characterised the homosexual epidemic, while sub-type C, common to the north of South Africa's borders, has characterised the heterosexual epidemic (Van Harmelen et al., 1997). By the early nineties the heterosexual epidemic had overtaken the homosexual epidemic in terms of numbers of new infections, and has since then been the main focus of public attention.

Numerous other sub-epidemics can be observed, particularly in the different race groups and the different provinces. To understand how the epidemic has evolved, it is necessary to appreciate the factors with which differentials in HIV prevalence are associated.

### Racial differentials

Currently income is distributed unevenly between the four race groups. The Human Development Index for the black African population is 0.5 – this compares with indices of 0.66 for coloureds, 0.84 for Asians, and 0.9 for whites (Department of Health and Population Development, 1998). The average black person earns a mere 13 per cent of what the average white person earns. Prevalence differentials between the race groups can thus be explained to some extent by the correlation between income and HIV prevalence.

The AIDS epidemic is most severe in the black population. The low income levels in the black population have been cited as a reason (Heywood, 1998), but the social effects of forced removals, the migrant labour system and the gradual breakdown of traditional society are also responsible. Much of the liberation movement involved the militarisation of black society and 'making the townships ungovernable' (Whiteside and Sunter, 2000), and has thus led to a disintegration of sexual mores and traditional values. Cultural differences in sex behaviour may also be the cause of the higher prevalence in the black population (dry sex, for example, is practised mostly among blacks).

Even among applicants for life assurance it has been suggested that HIV prevalence levels could be as much as ten times higher for blacks than for other races (Solomon, 1996). Prevalence levels in the general black population can be estimated from annual national antenatal clinic data (though there are various biases inherent in these surveys, as Missen (1998) observes). Figure 2.2 shows the trend in prevalence levels in the population of black females attending public antenatal clinics in the early years of the epidemic, when results were still stratified by race.

The closeness of the two curves can be attributed to the large percentage of the population that is black (76 per cent), and the relatively high fertility rates for black females (Department of Health and Population Development, 1998). As has been mentioned before, over 80 per cent of all pregnant women, of whom over 85 per cent are black African, attend public sector antenatal clinics (Department of Health, 2001).

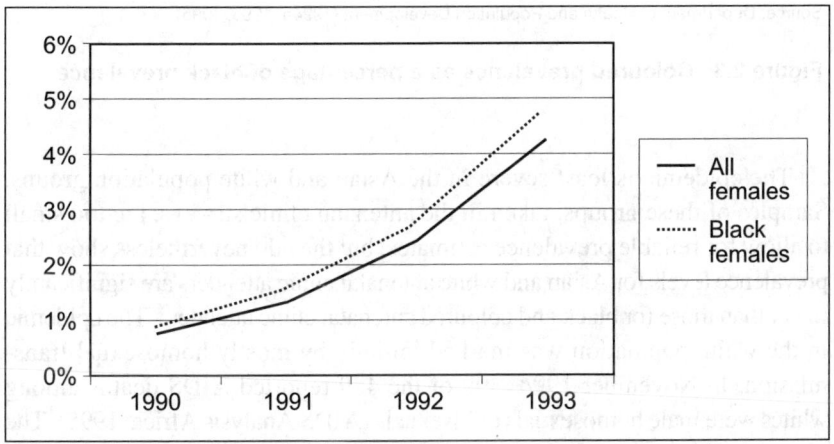

Source: Department of Health and Population Development (1994a)

**Figure 2.2 Prevalence levels amongst black antenatal clinic attenders.**

The epidemic in the coloured community is less severe. It is currently lagging the black epidemic, as is demonstrated by the rising HIV prevalence among coloureds relative to blacks (indicating a less mature epidemic in the coloured population). Figure 2.3 (based on data from the 1991–1995 antenatal clinic surveys) demonstrates this. Although a time lag is clearly present it is unlikely, given the higher socio-economic status of the coloured population (in particular greater access to healthcare, as well as other cultural differences), that the epidemic will peak at as high a level as it will in the black population. The ASSA2000 model projects that the ratio of the prevalence in the coloured population to that in the black African population increases further before levelling off at about 50 per cent.

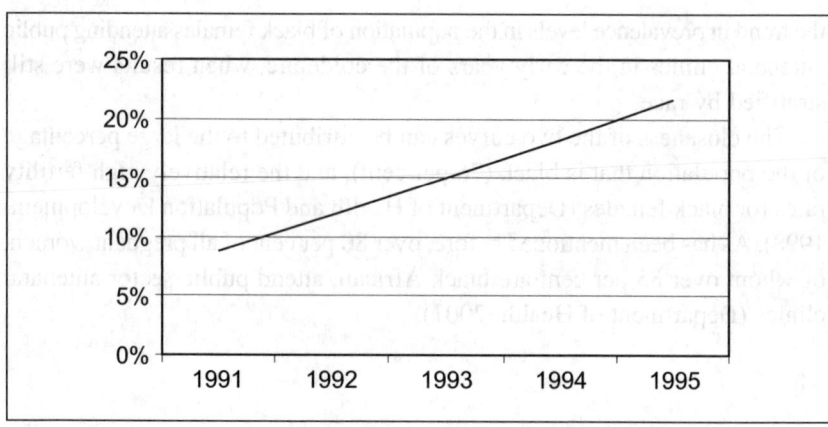

Source: Department of Health and Population Development (1994a, 1995, 1996)

**Figure 2.3  Coloured prevalence as a percentage of black prevalence.**

The epidemic is least severe in the Asian and white population groups. Samples of these groups, taken in the antenatal clinic surveys, are too small to allow for reliable prevalence estimates, but they do nevertheless show that prevalence levels for Asian and white antenatal clinic attenders are significantly lower than those for black and coloured antenatal clinic attenders. The epidemic in the white population was marked initially by mostly homosexual transmission. In November 1994, 399 of the 489 reported AIDS deaths among whites were male homosexuals or bisexuals (AIDS Analysis Africa, 1995). The extent to which the heterosexual epidemic will develop in the Asian and white populations is still very much a matter of conjecture.

**Gender differentials**

It is commonly believed that HIV prevalence levels are higher among women than men in a purely heterosexual epidemic. Women are biologically more susceptible to infection. With the income share of women being only 30.5 per cent of national income (Department of Health and Population Development, 1998), they are also more susceptible because of their lower socio-economic position. Many women are, as a result of their financial dependence on their partners, unable to insist on safer sexual practices.

In the early stages of the epidemic, estimates of male prevalence as a percentage of female prevalence usually fall between 67 per cent and 75 per cent, as Table 2.3 shows.

**Table 2.3  Male to female prevalence ratios.**

|  | Male/Female prevalence |
|---|---|
| Blood transfusion data 1986–1991 (Crookes and Heyns, 1992) | 0.68 |
| TB clinic attenders 1991–1994 (McAnerney, 1994) | 0.71 |
| Kustner et al., 1994 | 0.73 |
| Webb, 1994a | 0.73 |

The differential between male and female prevalence levels is, however, likely to change over time. When the Lite version of the ASSA2000 model was run, it was found that this ratio rose from 76 per cent in 1990, to 82 per cent in 1995 and 88 per cent in 2000, but then dropped to 84 per cent in 2005 and stabilised at around 82 per cent by 2010. Thus, while it may have been acceptable to assume a ratio of 0.75 in the early stages of the epidemic, it is clearly inappropriate to be using this ratio at the current time. The Department of Health, in extrapolating from antenatal clinic results to the general population, assumes a ratio of 0.85 (Department of Health, 2001).

It should also be recognised that although these ratios are fairly representative of the population as a whole, they do not apply in all sub-populations. McIntyre (1996) states that these prevalence ratios are likely to be closer to one in urban areas. In addition, blood transfusion data shows that while the above ratios typically apply to the black and coloured populations, the ratios in the Asian and white population groups are usually significantly greater than one (Abdool Karim et al., 1998; Crookes and Heyns, 1992). This undoubtedly reflects the significance of the Pattern I epidemic in these population groups.

**Age differentials**

Gender affects not only the general level of HIV prevalence, but also the shape of the prevalence curve as a function of age. The effect of age on HIV prevalence therefore needs to be discussed separately for men and women.

Among women, prevalence tends to peak between the ages of 20 and 25, with social and economic pressures encouraging high-risk sexual behaviour at early ages, particularly with men who are significantly older. In the teenage age-group, antenatal clinic data may be somewhat biased, as a relatively large proportion of the pregnancies in this age-group are likely to be unintended. In the older age-groups, antenatal clinic data (included in Appendix 2.1) shows a rising prevalence relative to the prevalence in the 20–25 age-group. This is illustrated in Figure 2.4.

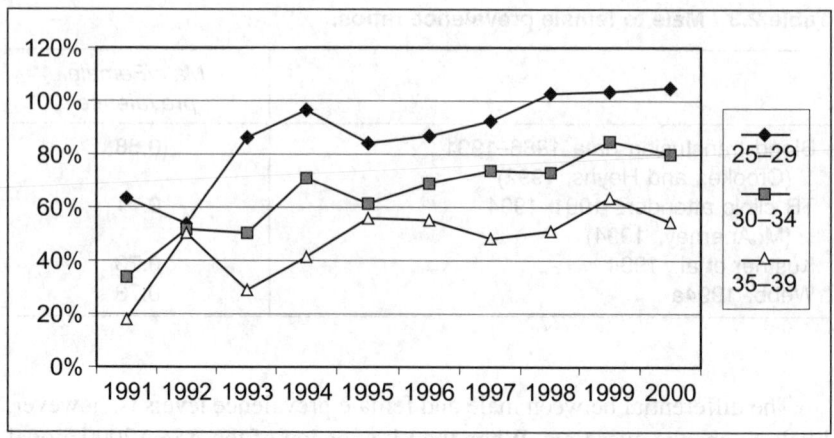

Source: Department of Health and Population Development (1995, 1996, 1997), Department of Health (1999, 2001)

**Figure 2.4 Prevalence relative to that of the 20–25 age group.**

This suggests that incidence drops off quite rapidly after the late teens and early twenties, with the high proportions surviving to later ages showing up significantly as the epidemic matures. The antenatal clinic data does not provide reliable prevalence estimates for women over the age of 40, but data from tuberculosis patients (biased though it is) suggests that even among women between the ages of 40 and 60 prevalence (at around 20 per cent) may remain quite high (McAnerney, 1994).

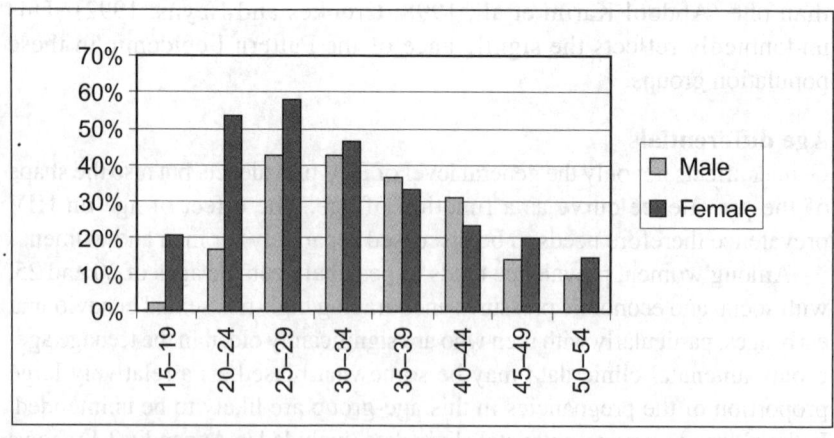

Source: Williams et al. (2000b)

**Figure 2.5 HIV prevalence by age and gender in Carletonville.**

In men, HIV prevalence tends to peak later (usually between the ages of 30 and 35), and at lower levels. The following age prevalence curves were determined by Williams et al. (2000b) in their study of men and women in Carletonville, and provide an example of how prevalence levels vary by age and gender.

**Geographical spread**

Early antenatal clinic data (see Appendix 2.1) suggests that the heterosexual epidemic began in KwaZulu-Natal. The epidemics in the other provinces appeared to lag behind the epidemic in KwaZulu-Natal, and Williams and Campbell (1998) have estimated these time lags (in years) to be as shown in Figure 2.6.

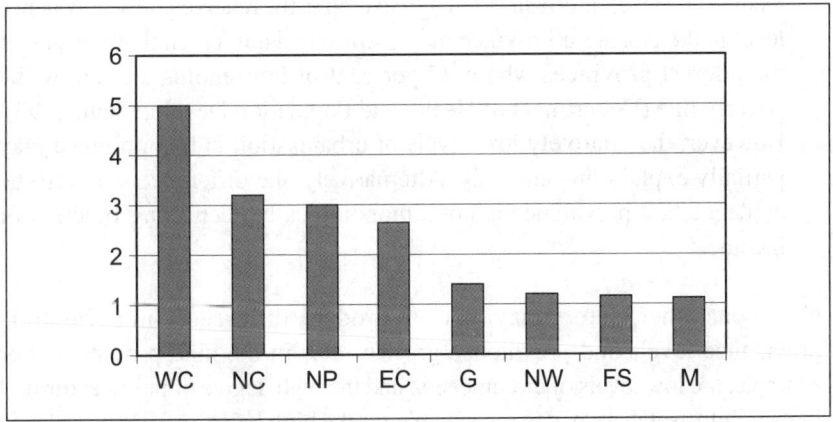

Source: Williams and Campbell (1998)

**Figure 2.6 Time lags between provincial epidemics and the epidemic in KwaZulu-Natal.**

These figures, however, are calculated on the assumption that the intrinsic growth rate and the asymptotic prevalence are the same for all nine provinces. Dorrington (2000) shows that while this may be a reasonable assumption for five of the provinces, it is not reasonable for KwaZulu-Natal, the Northern Province, the Northern Cape and the Western Cape. The following are some of the reasons why it may not be appropriate to fit a simple lag for the provinces.

- HIV prevalence levels are significantly higher in the black population than in other race groups, and there are likely to be corresponding differences

in peak prevalence levels. The proportion of the population that is black is relatively low in the Western Cape and Northern Cape, and this is likely to translate into lower peak prevalence rates in these provinces.
- The epidemic spreads more quickly to, and is most pervasive in, areas surrounding heavily-travelled roads. Wawer et al. (1997) show that in Uganda prevalence is highest in main road trading centres (31 per cent), second highest in trading villages (23 per cent), and lowest in agrarian villages off main and secondary roads (13 per cent). This is partly due to through roads between large towns and cities attracting sex worker interaction with truckers and travellers. The fact that most of the trucking routes from the north terminate in Durban may explain why the epidemic has been slow to spread to the western half of the country (Webb, 1994b).
- Differences in prevalence levels can also be explained by differences in income and level of urbanisation. For example, the relatively low prevalence level in the Northern Province may seem surprising given that it is one of the poorest provinces where 77 per cent of households are below the poverty line (Department of Health and Population Development, 1998). However, the relatively low levels of urbanisation in this province may partially explain this anomaly. Alternatively, the difference may also be evidence that prevalence is not a monotonically decreasing function of income.

Numerous other factors may work to produce differences in asymptotic prevalence levels and prevalence growth rates in the nine provinces. For example, the low levels of circumcision and the high degree of political turmoil in KwaZulu-Natal are partly responsible for the high levels of HIV prevalence in this province.

**Urban–rural differentials**
Little investigation has been conducted locally into the difference between urban and rural levels of HIV prevalence. Early figures from the Johannesburg City Health Department suggested an urban prevalence roughly 2.7 times higher than the rural prevalence (Webb, 1994a). McAnerney (1994) reported, apparently for 1994, an antenatal clinic prevalence in rural areas of 2.5 per cent and a prevalence in urban areas of 9.4 per cent (about 3.8 times higher than for rural areas).

The fact that prevalence is lower in rural communities may seem surprising, given that levels of income and levels of knowledge about HIV/AIDS are lower in these regions. Furthermore, levels of prevalence of other sexually transmitted infections are higher in rural areas than in urban areas; for example, 9.1 per cent of men in urban areas report having had painful urination or discharges, or genital sores, in the last three months, while the corresponding proportion for non-urban areas was 16.6 per cent (Department of Health, 1999b). The explanation for the low prevalence levels in rural areas may lie in the limited scope for sexual networking in isolated communities, as well as the greater influence of traditional practices.

The urban–rural differential may also be due to temporal factors. In many sub-Saharan countries the AIDS epidemic has been slow to spread to rural communities because of their relative immobility and geographic isolation. Once the epidemic is imported into the rural community, the incidence pattern may follow that in urban areas – that is to say, the observed urban–rural differential may be due to a time lag. Chin and Sato (1994) suggest that as the epidemic spreads and as prevalence levels in urban areas begin to level off, the difference between urban and rural prevalence levels is likely to diminish. The ratios quoted in the first paragraph will therefore decline with time.

If this is indeed a valid explanation of urban–rural differentials in sub-Saharan Africa, it should not be assumed that the same factors will work to produce an urban–rural differential in South Africa. Rural communities in this country are not as static or as geographically isolated as those in the rest of Africa. The migrant labour system has caused a steady flow of HIV-infected men into and out of the rural communities in which their wives and families are situated, and the urban areas in which they work. The superior transport system in South Africa may also have ensured a more rapid spread of the epidemic to rural areas. Piot et al. (1994) have noted that in Côte d'Ivoire (a country which, like South Africa, has good road and transport systems) HIV has spread equally into urban and rural areas (but at a much lower level). That the differential should be relatively small in South Africa is confirmed by one of the country's few sentinel surveys: Wilkinson et al. (1999b) show that the prevalence levels in Hlabisa, a rural district in KwaZulu-Natal, initially lagged behind those of the province as a whole but appear to have caught up more recently.

## *The model*

The projections in this chapter are based on the ASSA2000 suite of models developed by the Actuarial Society of South Africa. These models have their origin in a proprietary model, the Metropolitan-Doyle model, first developed in 1989 (Doyle and Millar, 1990) but have developed independently of this model since 1993. The early version of the ASSA model, the ASSA500 modelled the impact of the epidemic on a hypothetical population, and was useful mainly for illustration and experimentation. This was followed by the currently publicly available model (the ASSA600) which attempted to model the impact of the epidemic on the South African population as a whole, and as such was an AIDS and demographic model (Dorrington, 1998).

ASSA2000 is a component population projection model that models the demographic impact of the heterosexual (Pattern II) epidemic. The model splits the population into various risk groups according to the mode and probability of becoming infected, as follows:

- By age, with the young (0–13 years old) becoming infected only via their mothers, the adults (14–59) becoming infected by heterosexual intercourse, and the old (over 59) who are infected only by past indiscretions.
- By behaviour, with a small percentage (around one per cent) being commercial sex workers and their regular clients, a larger percentage (around 20 per cent) being those regularly infected with STDs, a major co-factor in the spread of the epidemic, a larger percentage (around 40 per cent) being those who practice risky sexual intercourse but are not infected with STDs, and a similar proportion who are not at risk.
- By socio-cultural and economic status, for which population group is used as a proxy.
- By geographic area, for which province is used as a proxy.

The suite comprises the ASSA2000 model which takes into account race, the Lite model which models the population as a whole irrespective of race and then the application of the ASSA2000 model to each of the provinces, which when aggregated probably provides the most reliable estimate of the demographic impact in South Africa.

Unfortunately the ASSA2000 suite of models are not yet fully calibrated (to fit past data) because, despite the promise of more detailed provincial-level data four months of fairly persistent enquiry has not managed to ensure delivery. Thus the results presented here are tentative in that final calibration may lead to some fine-tuning. However, it is not expected that the overall patterns will be very different.

## The projections

Table 2.4 Comparison of past prevalences from the model with those from the antenatal clinic survey.

|  | 1990 | 1991 | 1992 | 1993 | 1994 | 1995 | 1996 | 1997 | 1998 | 1999 | 2000 |
|---|---|---|---|---|---|---|---|---|---|---|---|
| Population | 0.1% | 0.3% | 0.6% | 1.1% | 1.8% | 2.9% | 4.5% | 6.3% | 8.2% | 10.1% | 11.7% |
| Adults (15+) | 0.2% | 0.4% | 0.9% | 1.6% | 2.8% | 4.4% | 6.6% | 9.2% | 12.0% | 14.6% | 16.9% |
| Women 15–49 | 0.3% | 0.6% | 1.2% | 2.2% | 3.7% | 5.9% | 8.7% | 12.0% | 15.4% | 18.7% | 21.5% |
| Antenatal clinic survey | 0.8% | 1.4% | 2.4% | 4.3% | 7.6% | 10.4% | 14.2% | 17.0% | 22.8% | 22.4% | 24.5% |

As can be seen from Table 2.4 estimates of prevalence based on the annual antenatal survey have been higher than those of all women in the child bearing age-range, which in turn are higher than those of all adults, which in turn are higher than those for the population as a whole. The excess of the ANC prevalence above that of all women 15–49 in the more recent years (and into the future) is due to the fact that the distribution of women attending antenatal clinics by age is becoming increasingly different from that of the general population as HIV impacts on fertility of the older women. In the earlier years, however, the difference reflects a probable bias in the antenatal surveys, probably due to a concentration of the sample clinics in the urban areas (at a time when the prevalence in the urban areas was significantly greater than that in the rural areas, which is much less the case today). It may be assumed that most of this bias had disappeared by 1998 (when the new protocol was introduced).

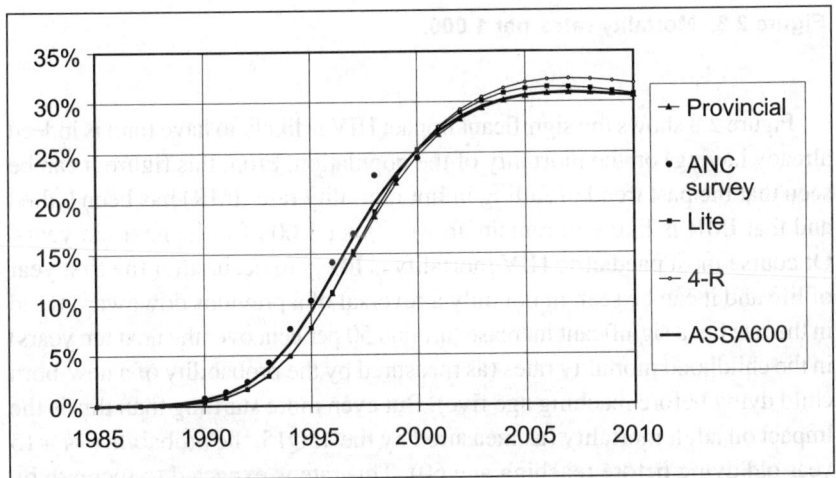

**Figure 2.7  Projections of the various models compared to the antenatal clinic survey results.**

Figure 2.7 compares the projections of the various ASSA2000 models with the ANC survey results. Included for continuity is the projection from the previous model, the ASSA600. From this comparison it can clearly be seen how the ASSA2000 models have been adjusted to allow for the assumed bias in the early ANC results, but that all versions of the model suggest that the expected prevalence at ANC clinics will have reached between 31 and 32 per cent by 2010.

## 36 Impacts and Interventions

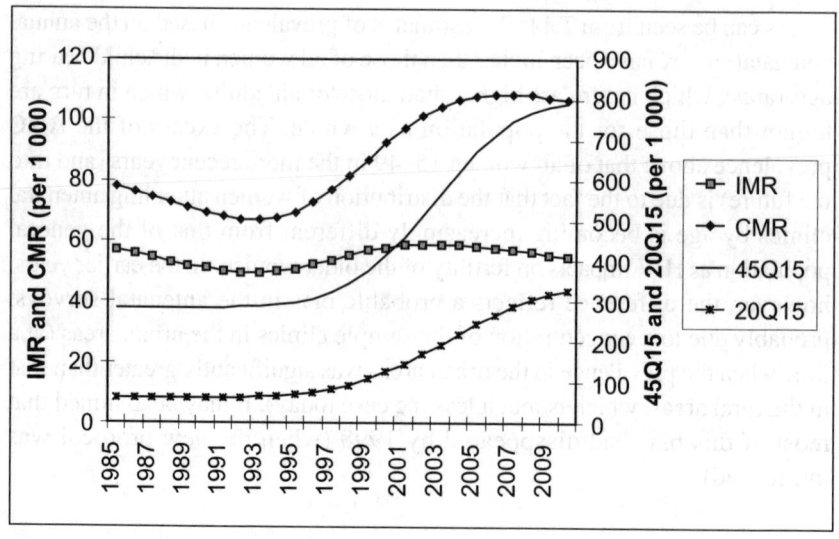

**Figure 2.8** Mortality rates per 1 000.

Figure 2.8 shows the significant impact HIV is likely to have (and is indeed already having) on the mortality of the population. From this figure it can be seen that the past trend of falling infant mortality rate (IMR) has been halted and that IMR is likely to remain above 50 per 1 000 for the next ten years. Of course most paediatric HIV mortality is likely to occur after the first year of life and it can be seen in not only a reversal of a previous downward trend in the rate but a significant increase (around 50 per cent over the next ten years) in the childhood mortality rates (as measured by the probability of a new-born child dying before reaching age five). But even more startling than this is the impact on adult mortality (as measured by the 45Q15, the probability of a 15 year old dying before reaching age 60). This rate is expected to increase by around 150 per cent by 2010, from 30 per cent to 80 per cent, implying that without behavioural change and interventions half the adult population can be expected to contract the virus during their life times.

As shown in Figure 2.9 these effects have the consequence of reducing the life expectancy at birth from over 60 years in the mid-1990s to slightly above 40 by 2010.

Epidemiological and Demographic 37

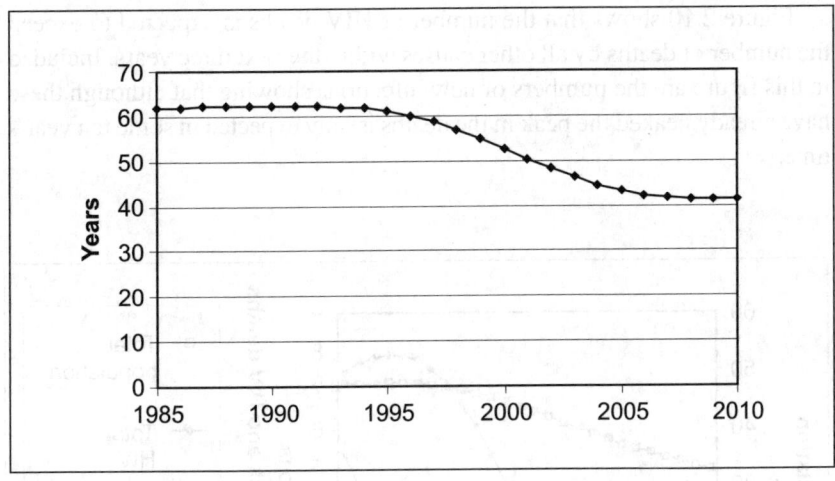

**Figure 2.9** The impact on the life expectancy at birth.

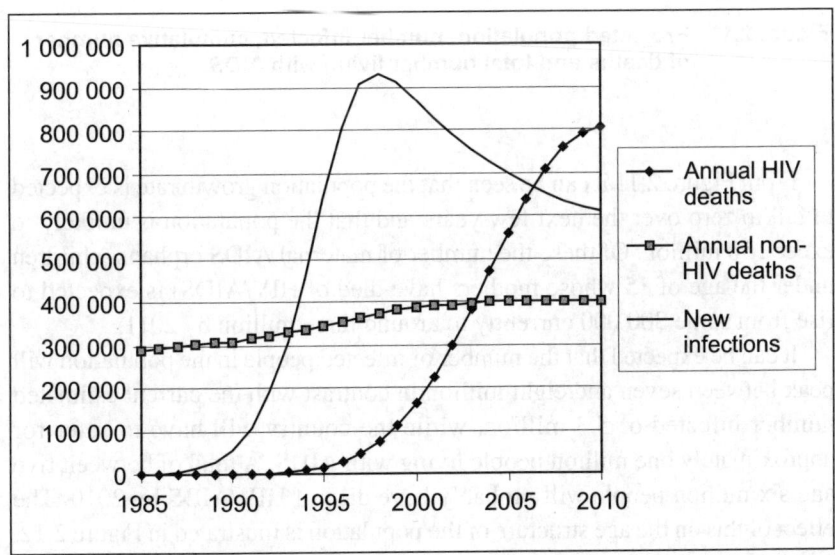

**Figure 2.10** Comparison of the number of new infections with the number of deaths.

Figure 2.10 shows that the number of HIV deaths is expected to exceed the number of deaths by all other causes within the next three years. Included in this figure are the numbers of new infections showing that although these have already peaked the peak in the deaths is only expected in some ten year's time.

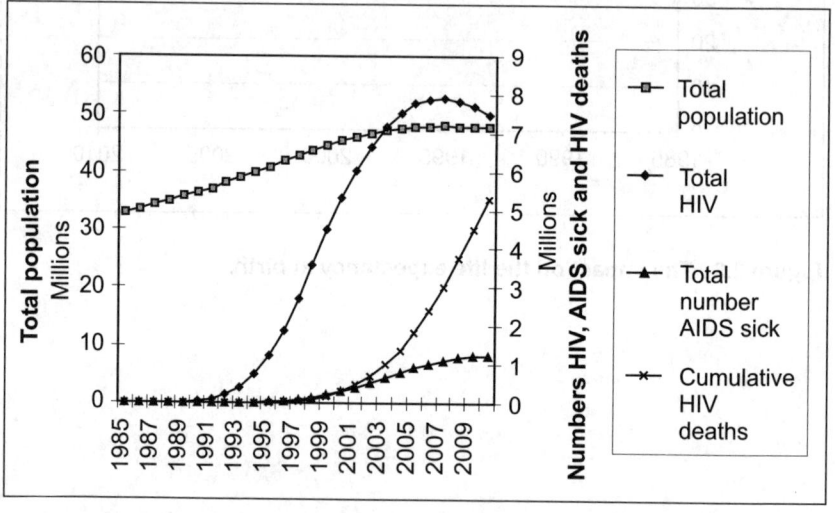

**Figure 2.11** Projected population, number infected, cumulative number of deaths and total number living with AIDS.

From Figure 2.11 it can be seen that the population growth rate is expected to fall to zero over the next few years and that the population is unlikely to exceed 50 million. Of these the number of maternal AIDS orphans (children under the age of 15 whose mothers have died of HIV/AIDS) is expected to rise from some 300 000 currently to around three million by 2011.

It can be expected that the number of infected people in the population will peak between seven and eight million in contrast with the current estimated number infected of 5.3 million, while the country will have to cater for approximately one million people living with AIDS. A total of between five and six million people will probably have died of HIV/AIDS by 2010. The effect of this on the age structure of the population is illustrated in Figure 2.12, where the outer line represents the pyramid expected in 2010 had there not been an HIV/AIDS epidemic and the solid pyramid is expected as a result of the epidemic.

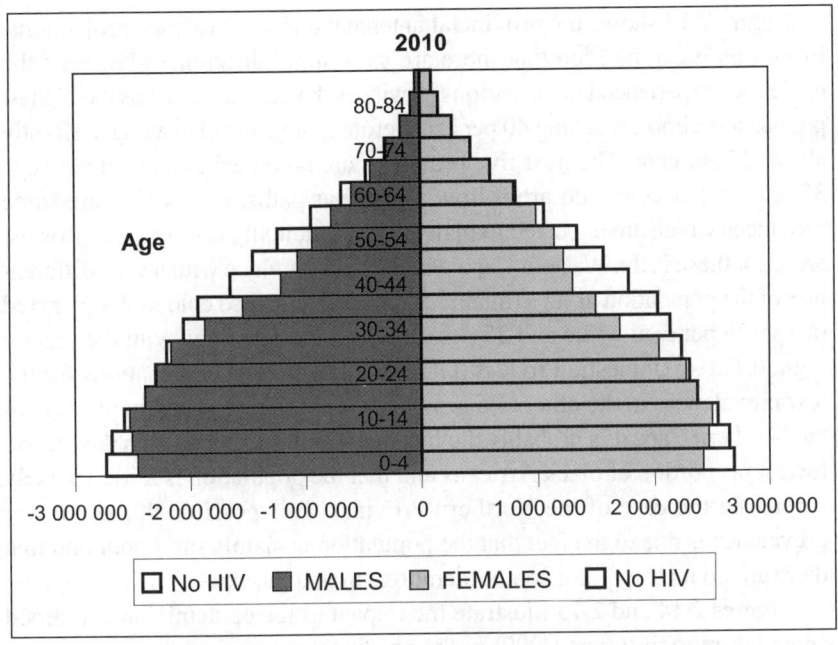

**Figure 2.12** Population pyramid in mid-2010 showing the impact of HIV/AIDS on the total population.

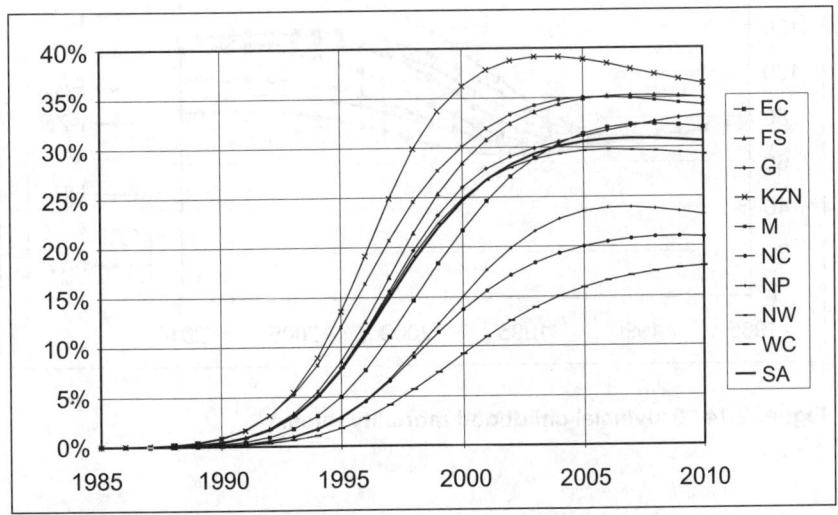

**Figure 2.13** Provincial antenatal clinic prevalence projections.

Figure 2.13 shows the provincial antenatal clinic prevalence projections. From this it can be seen that there are substantial differences between the epidemics experienced in the various provinces. KwaZulu-Natal has the highest prevalence, almost reaching 40 per cent before falling and plateauing at slightly above 35 per cent. The next five provinces are predicted to plateau between 30 and 35 per cent, and are following similar paths. Below that are three provinces which are expected to plateau at substantially lower levels. Lowest amongst these is the Western Cape which is the province with a very different mix of the population groups (mainly 50 per cent so-called coloured (i.e. mixed races), 25 per cent white and 25 per cent black African) and with the second highest Gross Domestic Product (GDP) per capita. The explanations for the low prevalences in the other two provinces is not that clear but in the case of the Northern Cape it is probably the fact that it is the province with the second lowest proportion of black Africans and that the population is fairly sparsely spread. In the case of the Northern Province, it is possible that the lower prevalence is due to the fact that the population is mainly rural poor and that there are no metropolitan conglomerations in that province.

Figures 2.14 and 2.15 illustrate the impact of the epidemic on childhood and adult mortality (per 1 000) in the provinces respectively.

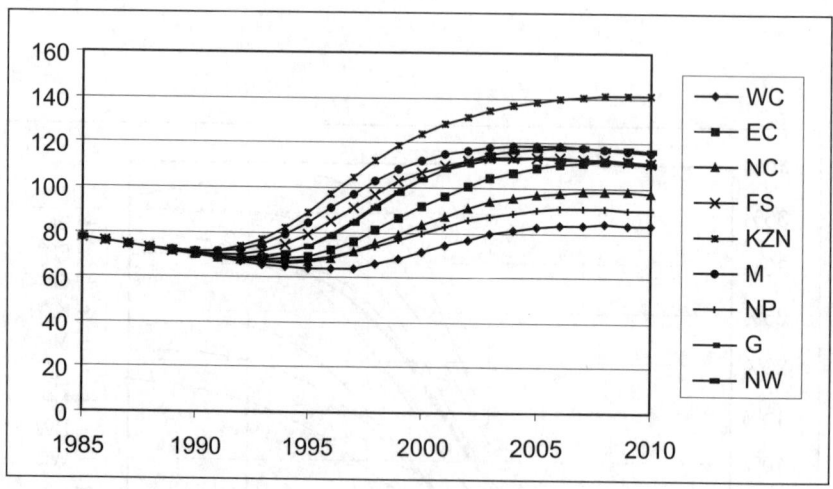

Figure 2.14 Provincial childhood mortality rates.

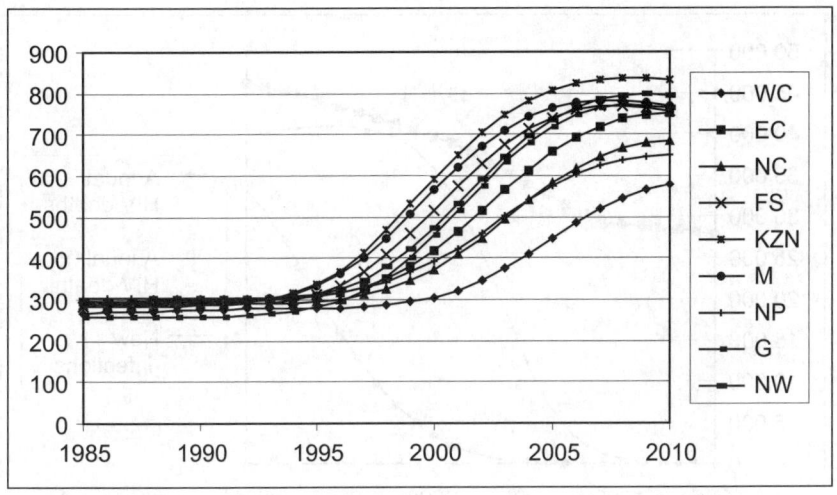

**Figure 2.15** Provincial adult mortality rates.

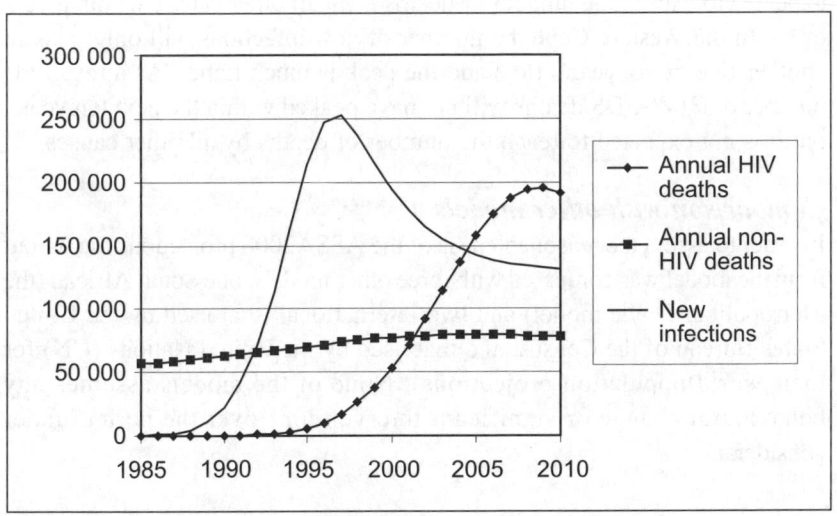

**Figure 2.16** Comparison of the number of new infections with the number of deaths in KwaZulu-Natal.

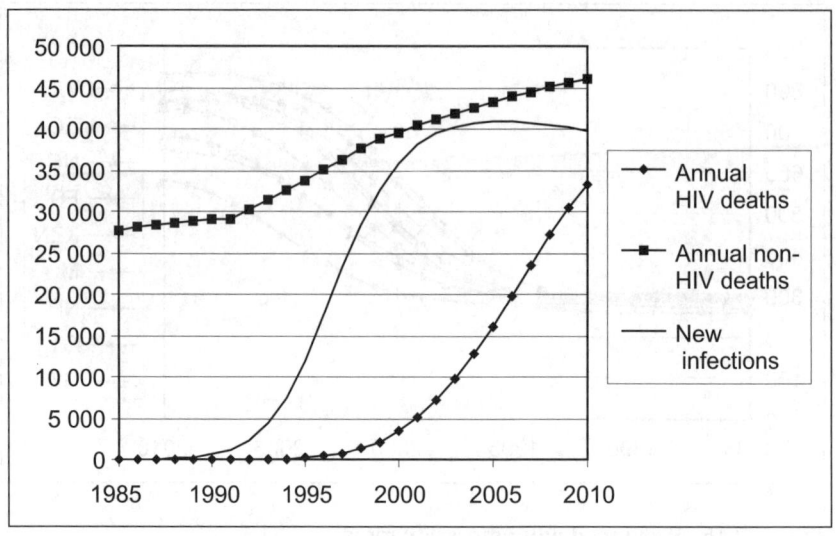

**Figure 2.17** Comparison of the number of new infections with the number of deaths in the Western Cape.

Figures 2.16 and 2.17 show the two extremes of the impact on deaths in provinces. In KwaZulu-Natal the number of new cases peaked in 1997 and since then has dropped off steeply and the number of HIV/AIDS deaths is expected to exceed the number of deaths from all other causes within a year or so. In the Western Cape the number of new infections will only peak in another five or six year's time and the peak is much flatter. As a result the number of HIV/AIDS deaths will not have peaked within the next ten years, but it is not expected to reach the number of deaths by all other causes.

## Comparison with other models

In order to assess the reasonableness of the ASSA2000 projections the output from the model was compared with three other models, one South African (the Metropolitan-Doyle model) and two international (that used by the United States Bureau of the Census, and that used by the United Nations (UN) for their world population projections). None of the models assumes any behavioural change or significant interventions over the period under consideration.

## Balance equations

The balance equations of the four models between the years 2000 and 2010 are presented in Table 2.5. From this comparison it can be seen that the models differ significantly in terms of the base population estimate. In particular, the UN estimate for the year 2000 is below the 1996 Census estimate, which itself is thought by many demographers to be an underestimate. The level of migration assumed also differs significantly (with, in particular, the United States Bureau of the Census assuming net out migration). These differences in migration undoubtedly explain a large part of the difference in the mid-year population estimates.

Table 2.5  Balance equations (figures in thousands).

|  | United States Bureau of the Census | United Nations | Metropolitan-Doyle | ASSA2000 |
|---|---|---|---|---|
| Mid-year population 2000 | 43 421 | 40 377 | 42 719 | 45 347 |
| +Births | 8 327 | 10 125 | 9 573 | 10 947 |
| −Deaths: non-AIDS | 3 173 | 2 598 | 3 911 | 3 965 |
| −Deaths: AIDS | 6 999 | 5 402 | 3 755 | 4 991 |
| +Net immigration | −468 | 13 | 0 | 313 |
| Mid-year population 2010 | 41 108 | 42 515 | 44 626 | 47 651 |

In order to better compare the models the figures were recast assuming the same base population and level of migration as the ASSA2000 model (Table 2.6). From these figures the following observations are made:

- The impact of HIV/AIDS is projected to be significant (between four and seven million deaths in the next ten years).
- Non-AIDS deaths in the Metropolitan-Doyle model appear to be too high.
- AIDS deaths from both the United Nations and the United States Bureau of the Census models appear to be too high.
- UN births appear to be too high (which might explain why they don't project a drop in population despite projecting quite high deaths) while births in the United States Bureau of the Census model appear to be on the low side.

**Table 2.6 Recast of balance equations to ASSA2000 base population and migration (figures in thousands).**

|  | United States Bureau of the Census | United Nations | Metropolitan-Doyle | ASSA2000 |
|---|---|---|---|---|
| Mid-year population 2000 | 46 079 | 46 079 | 46 079 | 45 347 |
| +Births | 9 502 | 13 278 | 11 196 | 10 947 |
| −Deaths: non-AIDS | 3 621 | 3 407 | 4 574 | 3 965 |
| −Deaths: AIDS | 7 987 | 7 084 | 4 391 | 4 991 |
| +Net immigration | 313 | 313 | 313 | 313 |
| Mid-year population 2010 | 44 287 | 49 179 | 48 622 | 47 651 |

Figures in italics have been estimated by the authors

## Comparison of the estimates of the impact of HIV/AIDS

Table 2.7 compares various HIV/AIDS-related output of the models (where available) for the years 2000 and 2010. From this notice the following:

- The models all project a significant increase in mortality and a drop in life expectancy of between five and 16 years over the next ten years.
- The prevalence from the Metropolitan model, particularly, in the oldest age-groups appears to be too low.
- According to the United States Bureau of the Census model there have already been over a million AIDS deaths, which seems unlikely (particularly given that the ASSA2000 model is calibrated on the mortality data).
- The United States Bureau of the Census estimates for child mortality look completely out of line with the estimates from the other models.
- As does the United States Bureau of the Census's estimate that nearly a quarter of the total population will be HIV-positive by 2010, with over 50 per cent of the 30–44 year olds being infected.
- As a consequence their estimate of life expectancy of 35 years seems too low (while the United Nations' estimate of 46 years is probably on the high side).

Epidemiological and Demographic 45

Table 2.7 Comparison of output of the models (figures in thousands).

| 2000 | Total HIV | Total HIV (recast) | HIV Prevalence | | | | | Mortality | | | | |
|---|---|---|---|---|---|---|---|---|---|---|---|---|
| | | | Total | 15–29 | 30–44 | 45–59 | Deaths to date | IMR | Child Q5 | Adult 45Q15 | Life exp |
| ASSA2000 | 5 310 | 5 310 | 12% | 17% | 26% | 9% | 296 | 58 | 92 | 413 | 56 |
| Metropolitan | 3 755 | 3 986 | 9% | 21% | 14% | 1% | 352 | 60 | 97 | | 55 |
| US Bureau of the Census | 5 578 | 5 825 | 13% | 21% | 25% | 15% | 1 043 | 59 | 120 | 498 | 51 |
| UN | 4 332 | 4 583 | 11% | n/a | n/a | n/a | 1 069 | 61 | 96 | n/a | 51 |

| 2010 | Total HIV | Total HIV (recast) | HIV Prevalence | | | | | Mortality | | | | |
|---|---|---|---|---|---|---|---|---|---|---|---|---|
| | | | Total | 15–29 | 30–44 | 45–59 | Deaths to date | IMR | Child Q5 | Adult 45Q15 | Life exp |
| ASSA2000 | 7 487 | 7 487 | 16% | 23% | 33% | 15% | 5 287 | 55 | 106 | 791 | 40 |
| Metropolitan | 6 484 | 6 924 | 15% | 27% | 32% | 3% | 4 107 | 59 | 120 | | 39 |
| US Bureau of the Census | 10 135 | 11 748 | 25% | 32% | 53% | 35% | 8 042 | 67 | 147 | 840 | 35 |
| UN | 6 685 | 7 017 | 16% | n/a | n/a | n/a | 6 471 | 58 | 103 | n/a | 46 |

Figures in italics have been estimated by the author
n/a (Figures could not be supplied)

It is interesting to contrast the above mortality estimates with those recently published by the WHO. The WHO estimates for 1999 are:

- child mortality (Q5) of 76 per thousand (i.e. lower than any of the above estimates for 2000);
- adult mortality (45Q15) of 567 per thousand (i.e. higher than any of the above estimates for 2000);
- life expectancy of 48 (i.e. lower than any of the above estimates for 2000).

From these comparisons it can be seen that there is a tendency for the international models to exaggerate the impact of the epidemic relative to that predicted by the local models and although the ASSA2000 is not the most conservative of the local models the results of the model are at least as plausible as those from the other models.

## *The number of orphans*

One of the most tragic consequences of the HIV/AIDS epidemic is the huge number of children orphaned as a result of parents dying from AIDS. Many of these children are HIV-positive themselves – having been infected by their mothers either at birth or through breast milk.

Up to now the number of these orphans has been increasing quite slowly and from a low base – and hence has attracted relatively little attention to date. South Africa's AIDS epidemic is still in its early stages relative to other African countries, and the levels of orphanhood seen elsewhere in Africa have yet to be experienced in this country. As the epidemic matures and AIDS mortality increases, the number of orphans is predicted to rise dramatically.

The country will face significant costs in the long-term if the question of these orphans is not managed effectively – such costs include increased juvenile crime, reduced literacy, and increased economic burden on government. Many of these costs can be reduced if action is taken now. Models of community-based care must be further developed, and forms of government assistance to those caring for orphaned children must be expanded.

It is imperative that the number and profile of orphans expected in future be understood if successful strategies to provide and care for them are to be developed. A recent study (Johnson and Dorrington, 2001) has estimated the number of orphans using the ASSA2000 AIDS and Demographic model of the Actuarial Society of SA. The focus of this study was primarily on maternal orphans (those whose mothers have died), but it also estimated the numbers of dual orphans (children that have lost both parents) and paternal orphans.

The number of orphans is emerging as a massive challenge – and the time to act is now. To appreciate the impact and the long-term nature of the challenge, it is useful to consider the HIV/AIDS epidemic as a series of waves (Figure 2.18). The first wave – people newly infected with HIV (the incidence) – has already peaked (in about 1998), at about 930 000 infections a year. This is followed by the wave of prevalence (the total number of people infected with HIV), which is projected to peak in about 2006, at between seven and eight million infected. The next wave – the AIDS deaths – is expected to peak soon after this in about 2010, at about 800 000 deaths a year. That in turn will be followed by the wave of AIDS orphans which is expected to peak at about 1.85 million in around 2015. This clearly illustrates that the rise in orphans is one of the most tragic long-term consequence of the epidemic.

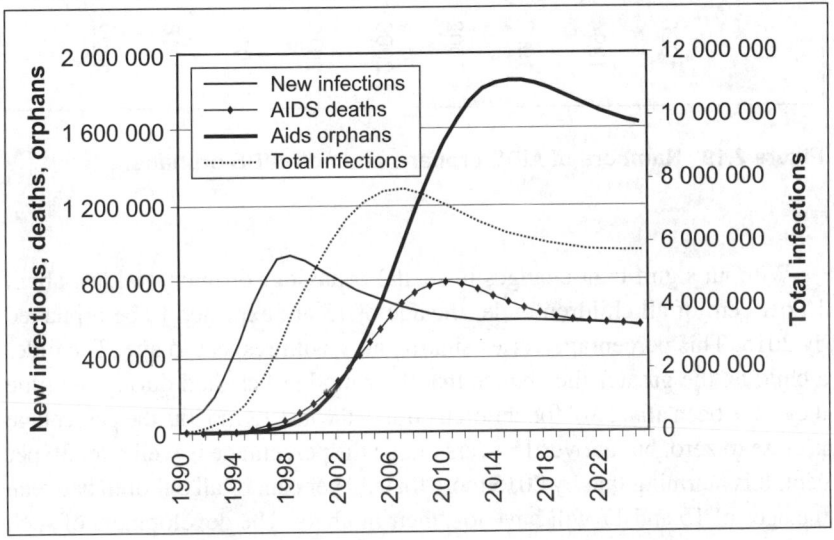

Figure 2.18  Waves of the AIDS epidemic.

It should be noted that HIV-positive orphans constitute a relatively small part of the orphan population, since about two-thirds of babies born to HIV-positive parents will not be infected, and because most infected children do not survive long enough to make up a sizeable proportion of the orphans.

Figure 2.19 shows numbers of AIDS orphans (those whose mothers died while HIV-positive) as against non-AIDS orphans (those whose mothers were HIV-negative) over time. Projections indicate that the number of non-AIDS orphans will gradually decline – mainly as a result of greater numbers of mothers dying from AIDS, and declining levels of fertility. However, the number of AIDS orphans is expected to rise enormously over the next decade, peaking at about 1.85 million in 2015.

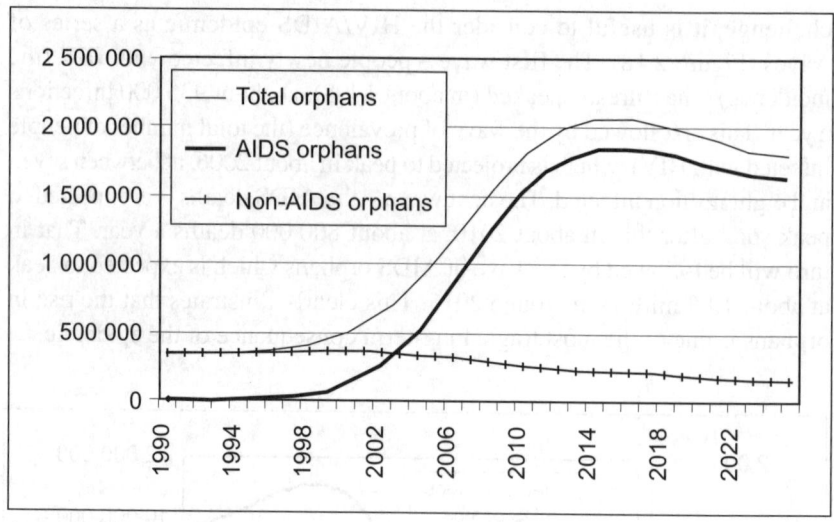

**Figure 2.19 Numbers of AIDS orphans and non-AIDS orphans.**

Without significant changes in sexual behaviour or interventions, about 15 per cent of all children under the age of 15 are expected to be orphaned by 2015. This percentage varies significantly with respect to age. The older a child is, the greater the chance that their mother has died during the time they have been alive. So, for children born in the last 12 months the percentage is close to zero, but at over 15 years of age the percentage is well over 30 per cent. It is alarming that by 2015 more than 30 per cent of all children between the ages of 15 and 17 will have lost their mothers. The development of such an orphan generation is likely to have profound effects on society.

Although the most commonly used definition of orphans is children under the age of 15 whose mothers have died, orphans do not cease to have need of parenting on reaching 15. The Constitution defines children as being persons under the age of 18, and most policymakers would agree that children under this age should not be expected to be self-supporting. Using age 18 as a cut-off results in a much higher estimate of orphans than using 15 years. The number of maternal orphans under the age of 18 is likely to peak at roughly 3.1 million in 2015, as opposed to 1.85 million using 15 years as cut-off. Apart from this the loss of a father can also have a significant impact.

On top of this, orphanhood may in practice begin long before the death of a parent. This will happen where there is a sole parent and that parent becomes sick with AIDS. Often the household is without income and the parent is no longer able to support the child. This and the trauma of watching the parent slowly dying are the first stresses the orphan has to face. Studies of AIDS orphans show that they have low self-esteem and tend to display more aggression, anxiety and depression than other children. Children alienated from or abandoned by their extended families are more likely to become street children and engage in antisocial behaviour or prostitution.

Regardless of the definition used, the number of orphans is likely to peak at around 2015 – at roughly two million in the case of maternal orphans under 15, and 3 million in maternal orphans under 18. The number of paternal orphans under 18 is expected to peak at 4.7 million in 2015, and the total number of children compromised by having lost one or both parents is likely to reach its highest level around 2015, at a staggering 5.7 million. The number of paternal and double orphans may be an underestimate of the number of children compromised, since it does not take into account fathers who are alive but absent (i.e. no longer taking responsibility for their children).

## Impact of mother-to-child-transmission prevention (MTCTP) programmes

In developed countries the probability of perinatal transmission of HIV can be reduced to very low levels through the provision of long-course anti-retroviral treatment during pregnancy and through Caesarean sections. In resource-poor settings it has been shown that giving short-course anti-retroviral treatment to mothers prior to birth and to babies after birth can also be effective in reducing the probability of transmission by between 35–50 per cent. It is often suggested that introducing a mother-to-child-transmission prevention (MTCTP) programme will result in a substantial increase in the numbers of orphans. Figure 2.20 shows the projected number of maternal orphans under the age of 15 if a MTCTP programme is introduced, compared to the levels expected if such a programme is not introduced. It is clear that if MTCTP was phased in, fewer children would be infected by their HIV-positive mothers, and hence children would survive for longer. By 2015 the number of orphans under 15 is likely to be around 2.26 million – 200 000 more than in the absence of MTCTP. Thus a MTCTP programme will only slightly increase the number of orphans, accounting for an additional ten per cent.

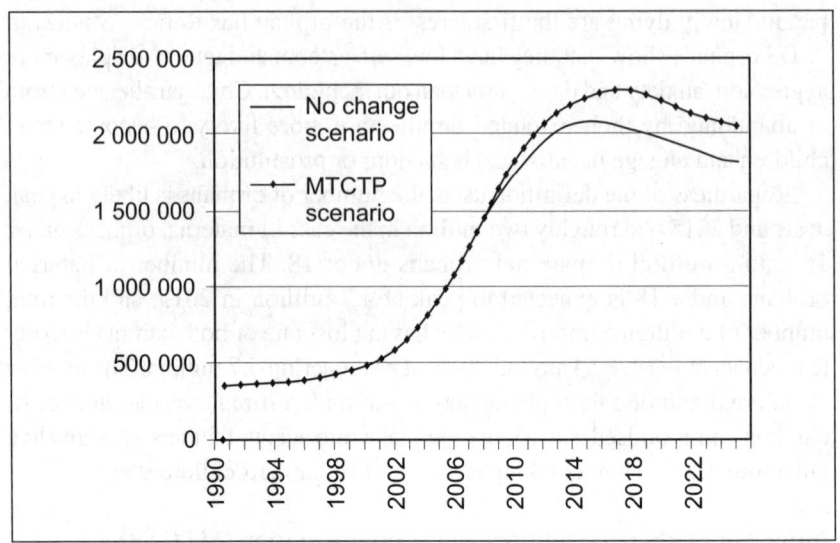

**Figure 2.20  Numbers of orphans, with and without an MTCTP programme.**

The expected number of orphans is – in the short term at least – relatively insensitive to changes in sexual behaviour patterns, condom distribution, AIDS awareness programmes, etc. These changes reduce the number of orphans substantially in the long term (by about ten per cent around 2015). However, such interventions are unlikely to change the fact that 12 years from now, there will be close to two million orphans.

Although prevention programmes may not achieve a short-term reduction in the number of orphans, a significant reduction in the number and trend in number of orphaned children can be achieved through anti-retroviral treatment programmes to all HIV-positive individuals. Such programmes may succeed in extending the lives of a large number of parents to the stage where their children are self-supporting. By 2015 the number of maternally orphaned children could be roughly half the number expected without any anti-retroviral intervention (Figure 2.21), at 1.15 million. The cost-effectiveness of such interventions needs to be assessed as a matter of urgency.

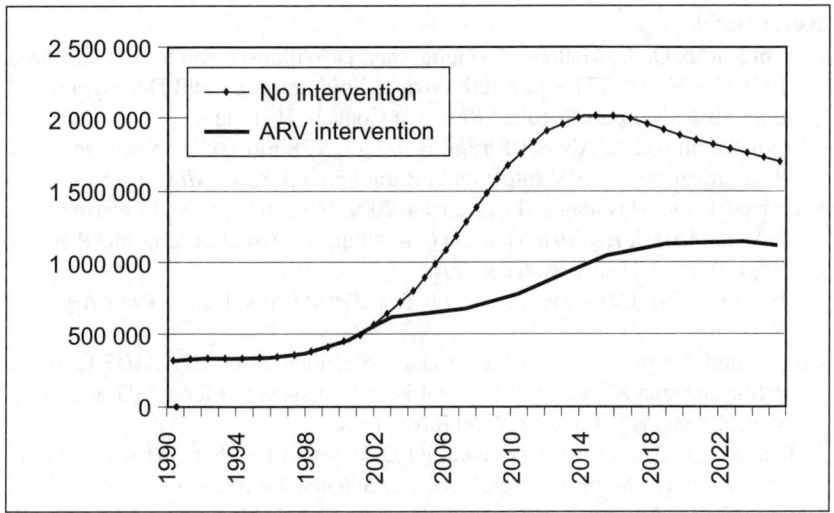

**Figure 2.21  Numbers of orphans, with and without anti-retroviral interventions.**

## Conclusion

That South Africa has experienced such a rapid spread of the HIV/AIDS epidemic should not have come as a surprise to anyone familiar with the conditions in this country prior to 1994. Apartheid left the country with all the ingredients to ensure that it would have the most explosive and extensive epidemic in the world. This, coupled with mismanagement of the epidemic at virtually every turn, has meant that the country is now facing a disaster which it barely comprehends.

Part of this mismanagement has been the failure to monitor properly the spread of the epidemic (for example the most recent official death data is for 1996). Data that is collected as part of the national antenatal seroprevalence survey is only made available at an aggregate level. Even then not all the data is published and researchers are expressly barred from access to the detailed data.

Of course, without detailed data it is not only impossible to understand the nature of the antenatal survey estimates, but it is also difficult to spot and interpret behavioural changes when they do occur. Although projecting the likely path of the epidemic under these conditions is difficult, past efforts to do so have been sadly accurate, and at the moment the epidemic seems to be following, blindly, the 'no behavioural change – no intervention' path.

## References

Abdool Karim, Q., C. Mathews, S. Gutmacher, D. Wilkinson and S. Abdool Karim. 1998. 'HIV and STDs in South Africa: Epidemiology and Demographics'. Unpublished Report, Medical Research Council, Pretoria.

Abdool Karim, Q., S. Abdool Karim, B. Singh, R. Short and S. Ngxongo. 1992. 'Seroprevalence of HIV Infection in Rural South Africa'. *AIDS* 6: 1535–1539.

Bradshaw, D., K. Masiteng and N. Nannan. 2001. 'Health Status and Determinants'. In *South African Health Review 2000*, A. Ntuli, N. Crisp, E. Clarke and P. Barron (eds). Durban: Health Systems Trust.

Caelers, D. 1999. 'Costs Mount as 1700 Test HIV Positive Daily'. *Cape Argus*. 15 November.

Chin, J. and P. Sato. 1994. 'Estimates and Projections of the HIV/AIDS Epidemic in Sub-Saharan Africa'. In *AIDS in Africa*, M. Essex, S. Mboup, P.J. Kanki and M.R. Kalengayi (eds). New York: Raven Press.

Colvin, M. 2000. 'Sexually Transmitted Diseases in Southern Africa: A Public Health Crisis'. *South African Journal of Science* 96: 335–339.

Colvin, M., Q. Abdool Karim and A. 'Hoosen. 1997. Management of Sexually Transmitted Diseases in Workplace Based Clinics in KwaZulu/Natal: Implications for HIV'. *South African Journal of Public Health* 87: 245–249.

Crookes, R. and A. Heyns. 1992. 'HIV Seroprevalence: Data Derived from Blood Transfusion Services'. *South African Medical Journal* 82: 484–485.

Crush, J. 1995. 'Mine Migrancy in the Contemporary Era'. In *Crossing Boundaries: Mine Migrancy in a Democratic South Africa*, J. Crush and W. James (eds). Cape Town: Institute for Democracy in South Africa and International Development Research Centre.

Department of Health. 1999a. *1998 National HIV Sero-Prevalence Survey Among Women Attending Public Antenatal Clinics in South Africa*. Pretoria.

Department of Health. 1999b. *South Africa Demographic and Health Survey 1998: Preliminary Report*. Pretoria.

Department of Health. 2001. *National HIV and Syphilis Sero-Prevalence Survey of Women Attending Public Antenatal Clinics in South Africa, 2000*. Pretoria.

Department of Health and Population Development. 1994a. 'Fourth National HIV Survey of Women Attending Antenatal Clinics, South Africa, Oct/Nov 1993'. *Epidemiological Comments* 21(4): 68–78.

Department of Health and Population Development. 1994b. 'AIDS in South Africa: Reported AIDS cases as on 30 December 1994'. *Epidemiological Comments* 21(12): 286.

Department of Health and Population Development. 1995. 'Fifth National HIV Survey in Women Attending Antenatal Clinics of the Public Health Services in South Africa, Oct/Nov 1994'. *Epidemiological Comments* 22(4): 90–100.

Department of Health and Population Development. 1996. 'Sixth National HIV Survey of Women Attending Antenatal Clinics of the Public Health Services in South Africa, Oct/Nov 1995'. *Epidemiological Comments* 23(1): 3–15.

Department of Health and Population Development. 1997a. 'Seventh National HIV Survey of Women Attending Antenatal Clinics of the Public Health Services in South Africa, Oct/Nov 1996'. *Epidemiological Comments* 23(2): 5–6.

Department of Health and Population Development. 1997b. Seventh National HIV Survey of Women Attending Antenatal Clinics of the Public Health Services, October/November 1996. *Epidemiological Comments* 23(2): 14–16.

Department of Health and Population Development. 1998. 'White Paper on Population Policy'. March. Online. (accessed December 2001). http://www.polity.org.za/govdocs/white_papers/popwp.html

Dorrington, R. 1998. 'ASSA600: An AIDS Model of the Third Kind?' *Transaction of the Actuarial Society of South Africa* 12(1): 99–153.

Dorrington, R. 1999. 'AIDS Then, Now, Tomorrow'. Paper presented at the 3rd African Population Conference, Durban, 6–10 December.

Dorrington, R. 2000. 'The ASSA2000 Suite of Models'. Paper presented at the Actuarial Society of South Africa Convention, Cape Town.

Doyle, P. and D. Millar. 1990. 'A General Description of an Actuarial Model Applicable to the HIV Epidemic in South Africa'. *Transactions of the Actuarial Society of South Africa* 8(2): 561–593.

Heywood, M. 1996. 'HIV/AIDS in the Southern African Mining Sector'. *AIDS Analysis Africa* 6(5): 5–6.

Heywood, M. 1998. 'How the Poor Die: HIV/AIDS and Poverty in South Africa'. Unpublished memorandum for the South African Human Rights Commission/Commission for Gender Equality/National NGO Coalition.

Humbridge, M. 1990. 'AIDS/HIV and Social Dislocation in Natal'. *AIDS Analysis Africa* 1(3): 6–8.

Ijsselmuiden, C., G. Padayachee, W. Mashaba, O. Martiny and H. van Staden. 1990. 'Knowledge, Beliefs and Practices Among Black Gold Miners Relating to Transmission of HIV and Other Sexually Transmitted Diseases'. *South African Medical Journal* 78: 520–523.

Johnson, L. and R. Dorrington. 2001. 'The Impact of HIV/AIDS on Orphanhood in South Africa: A Quantitative Analysis'. Monograph Number 4. Centre for Actuarial Research, University of Cape Town, Cape Town.

Johnson, L. and D. Budlender. 2002. 'HIV Risk Factors: A Review of the Demographic, Socio-economic, Biomedical and Behavioural Determinants of HIV Prevalence in South Africa'. Monograph Number 8. Centre for Actuarial Research, University of Cape Town, Cape Town.

Kaiser Family Foundation. 2001. *Hot Prospects, Cold Facts: Portrait of a Young South Africa*. Johannesburg: Lovelife.

Kinghorn, K. and M. Steinberg. 1998. *HIV/AIDS in South Africa: The Impacts and the Priorities*. Pretoria: Department of Health.

Kustner, H., J. Swanevelder and A. van Middelkoop. 1994. 'National HIV Surveillance: South Africa, 1990–1992'. *South African Medical Journal* 84: 195–200.

Lurie, M. 2000. 'Migration and AIDS in Southern Africa: A Review'. *South African Journal of Science* 96: 343–347.

Lurie, M., B. Williams, A. Sturm, G. Garnett, D. Mkaya-Mwamburi and S. Abdool Karim. 2000. 'HIV Discordance Among Migrant and Non-Migrant Couples in South Africa'. Paper presented at the 13th International AIDS Conference, Durban.

Lurie, M., A. Harrison, D. Wilkinson and S. Abdool Karim. 1997. 'Circular Migration and Sexual Networking in Rural KwaZulu/Natal: Implications for the Spread of HIV and Other Sexually Transmitted Diseases'. *Health Transition Review* Suppl. 3, 7: 15–24.

Maartens, G., R. Wood, E. O'Keefe and C. Byrne. 1997. 'Independent Epidemics of Heterosexual and Homosexual HIV in South Africa: Survival Differences'. *Quarterly Journal of Medicine* 90: 449–454.

Marks, S. 2001. 'The Spread of HIV/AIDS in South Africa: Historical Perspectives'. Keynote address at the AIDS in Context Conference, University of the Witwatersrand, Johannesburg, 4–7 April.

McAnerney, J. 1994. 'HIV Seroprevalence in TB patients'. *AIDS Bulletin* 3(3): 14–15.

McIntyre, J. 1996. 'HIV/AIDS in South Africa: A Relentless Progression?' *South African Medical Journal* 86: 27–28.

Medical Research Council. 1998. 'The National STD/HIV/AIDS Surveillance System'. A report prepared for the Directorate of Health Systems Research and Epidemiology, Department of Health, Pretoria.

Missen, P. 1998. 'Antenatal HIV Data Are Not So Biased'. *AIDS Analysis Africa* 8(4): 11.

Moses, S., J. Bradley, N. Nagelkerks and A. Ronald. 1990. 'Geographical Patterns of Male Circumcision Practices in Africa: Association with HIV Seroprevalence'. *International Journal of Epidemiology* 19: 693–697.

Pham-Kanter, G., M. Steinberg and R. Ballard. 1996. 'Sexually Transmitted Diseases in South Africa'. *Genitourinary Medicine* 72: 160–171.

Piot, P., J. Goeman and M. Laga. 1994. 'The Epidemiology of HIV and AIDS in Africa'. In *AIDS in Africa*, M. Essex., S. Mboup, P. Kanki and M. Kalengayi (eds). Raven Press. New York.

Potgieter, M. 2000. 'AIDS in Mpumalanga'. Paper presented at the Joint Population Conference, Port Elizabeth, 2–6 October.

Platzky, L. and C. Walker. 1985. *The Surplus People: Forced Removals in South Africa*. Johannesburg: Ravan Press.

Rape Crisis Cape Town. 2001. 'The Rape Crisis Website: Statistics'. Online. (accessed December 2001). www.rapecrisis.org.za/statistics

Rees, H., M. Beksinska, K. Dickson-Tetteh, R. Ballard and Y. Htun. 2000. 'Commercial Sex Workers in Johannesburg: Risk Behaviour and HIV Status'. *South African Journal of Science* 96: 283–284.

Schoub, B., A. Smith, S. Lyons, S. Johnson, D. Martin, G. McGillivray, G. Padayachee, S. Naidoo, E. Fisher and H. Hurwitz. 1988. 'Epidemiological Considerations of the Present Status and Future Growth of the AIDS Epidemic in South Africa'. *South African Medical Journal* 74: 153–157.

Shell, R. 2000. 'Trojan Horses: HIV/AIDS and Military Bases in Southern Africa'. Unpublished.

Sher, R. 1989. 'HIV Infection in South Africa, 1982–1988'. *South African Medical Journal* 76: 314–318.

Solomon, G. 1996. 'South African Actuarial Society Report Back on AIDS in South Africa'. *AIDS Scan* 8(1): 3–7.

Statistics South Africa. 2000. 'October Household Survey 1999'. Statistical Release PO317. Online. (accessed December 2001). http://www.statssa.gov.za/Statistical_Releases/Statistical_Releases.htm

Sturm, A., D. Wilkinson, N. Ndovela, S. Bowen and C. Connolly. 1998. 'Pregnant Women as a Reservoir of Undetected Sexually Transmitted Diseases in Rural South Africa: Implications for Disease Control'. *American Journal of Public Health* 88: 1243–1245.

UNAIDS. 2000. *Report on the Global HIV/AIDS Epidemic: June 2000*. Geneva: United Nations.

Van Harmelen, J., R. Wood, M. Lambrick, E. Rybicki, A. Williamson and C. Williamson. 1997. 'An Association Between HIV-1 Subtypes and Mode of Transmission in Cape Town, South Africa'. *AIDS* 11: 81–87.

Vundule, C., F. Maforah, R. Jewkes and E. Jordaan. 2001. 'Risk Factors for Teenage Pregnancy Among Sexually Active Black Adolescents in Cape Town'. *South African Medical Journal* 91: 73–80.

Wawer, M., D. Serwadda, R. Gray, N. Sewankambo, C. Li, F. Nalugoda, T. Lutalo and J. Konde-Lulu. 1997. 'Trends in HIV-1 Prevalence May Not Reflect Trends in Incidence in Mature Epidemics: Data from the Rakai Population-Based Cohort, Uganda'. *AIDS* 11: 1023–1030.

Webb, D. 1994a. 'Modelling the Emerging Geography of HIV'. *AIDS Analysis Africa* 4(4): 1–3.

Webb, D. 1994b. 'Mapping the AIDS pandemic: Geographical Progression of HIV in South Africa 1990–93'. *Nursing RSA* 9: 20–21.

Whiteside, A. and C. Sunter. 2000. *AIDS: The Challenge for South Africa*. Cape Town: Human & Rousseau and Tafelberg.

Wilkinson, D. 1999. 'HIV Infection Among Pregnant Women in the South African Private Medical Sector'. *AIDS* 13: 1783.

Wilkinson, D., S. Abdool Karim, A. Harrison, M. Lurie, M. Colvin, C. Connolly and A. Sturm. 1999a. 'Unrecognized Sexually Transmitted Infections in Rural South African Women: A Hidden Epidemic'. *Bulletin of the WHO* 77: 22–28.

Wilkinson, D., C. Connolly and K. Rotchford. 1999b. 'Continued Explosive Rise in HIV Prevalence Among Pregnant Women in Rural South Africa'. *AIDS* 13: 740.

Williams, B., D. Gilgen, C. Campbell, D. Taljaard and C. MacPhail. 2000a. *The Natural History of HIV/AIDS in South Africa: A Biomedical and Social Survey in Carletonville*. Johannesburg: Council for Scientific and Industrial Research.

Williams, B., E. Gouws, M. Colvin, F. Sitas, G. Ramjee and S. Abdool Karim. 2000b. 'Patterns of HIV Infection: Using Age Prevalence Data to Understand the Epidemic of HIV in South Africa'. *South African Journal of Science* 96: 305–312.

Williams, B. and C. Campbell. 1998. 'Understanding the Epidemic of HIV in South Africa'. *South African Medical Journal* 84: 247–251.

World Health Organisation. 2000. *The World Health Report 2000, Annexure 2*. Geneva: World Health Organisation.

Zwi, A. and D. Bachmayer. 1990. 'HIV and AIDS in South Africa: What Is An Appropriate Public Health Response?' *Health Policy and Planning* 5: 316–326.

Zwi, A. and A. Cabral. 1991. 'Identifying "High Risk Situations" for Preventing AIDS'. *British Medical Journal* 303: 1527–1529.

## Appendix 2.1 Results from antenatal clinic surveys

| Year | 1990 | 1991 | 1992 | 1993 | 1994 | 1995 | 1996 | 1997 | 1998 | 1999 | 2000 |
|---|---|---|---|---|---|---|---|---|---|---|---|
| National prevalence | 0.76% | 1.35% | 2.42% | 4.25% | 7.57% | 10.44% | 15.07% | 17.04% | 22.8% | 22.4% | 24.5% |
| **Age band** | | | | | | | | | | | |
| <20 | | 1.79% | 2.62% | 4.57% | 6.47% | 9.50% | 12.78% | 12.7% | 21.0% | 16.5% | 16.1% |
| 20–24 | | 2.15% | 3.92% | 6.06% | 8.94% | 13.12% | 17.52% | 19.7% | 26.1% | 25.6% | 29.1% |
| 25–29 | | 1.37% | 2.11% | 5.22% | 8.63% | 11.03% | 15.21% | 18.2% | 26.9% | 26.4% | 30.6% |
| 30–34 | | 0.72% | 2.04% | 3.05% | 6.37% | 8.05% | 12.13% | 14.5% | 19.1% | 21.7% | 23.3% |
| 35–39 | | 0.39% | 1.98% | 1.76% | 3.72% | 7.37% | 9.67% | 9.5% | 13.4% | 16.2% | 15.8% |
| 40–44 | | 0.95% | 0% | 2.44% | 5.28% | 4.36% | 9.94% | 7.5% | 10.5% | 12.0% | 10.2% |
| 45–49 | | 0% | 0% | 0% | 0.41% | 7.45% | 5.83% | 8.8% | 10.2% | 7.5% | 13.1% |
| **Province** | | | | | | | | | | | |
| KwaZulu-Natal | 1.61% | 2.86% | 4.50% | 9.53% | 14.35% | 18.23% | 19.90% | 26.9% | 32.5% | 32.5% | 36.2% |
| Mpumalanga | 0.38% | 1.21% | 2.23% | 2.40% | 12.16% | 16.18% | 15.77% | 22.6% | 30.0% | 27.3% | 29.7% |
| Free State | 0.59% | 1.50% | 2.86% | 4.12% | 9.19% | 11.03% | 17.49% | 20.0% | 22.8% | 27.9% | 27.9% |
| Northwest | 1.05% | 6.54% | 0.94% | 2.19% | 6.71% | 8.30% | 25.13% | 18.1% | 21.3% | 23.0% | 22.9% |
| Gauteng | 0.66% | 1.12% | 2.53% | 4.13% | 6.44% | 12.03% | 15.49% | 17.1% | 22.5% | 23.9% | 29.4% |
| Eastern Cape | 0.44% | 0.58% | 0.96% | 1.94% | 4.52% | 6.00% | 8.10% | 12.6% | 15.9% | 18.0% | 20.2% |
| Northern Province | 0.26% | 0.48% | 1.05% | 1.79% | 3.04% | 4.89% | 7.96% | 8.2% | 11.5% | 11.4% | 13.2% |
| Northern Cape | 0.20% | 0.12% | 0.65% | 1.07% | 1.81% | 5.34% | 6.47% | 8.6% | 9.9% | 10.1% | 11.2% |
| Western Cape | 0.06% | 0.08% | 0.25% | 0.56% | 1.16% | 1.66% | 3.09% | 6.3% | 5.2% | 7.1% | 8.7% |

Source: Department of Health and Population Development (1994, 1995, 1996, 1997), Department of Health (1999a, 2001)

*cont.*

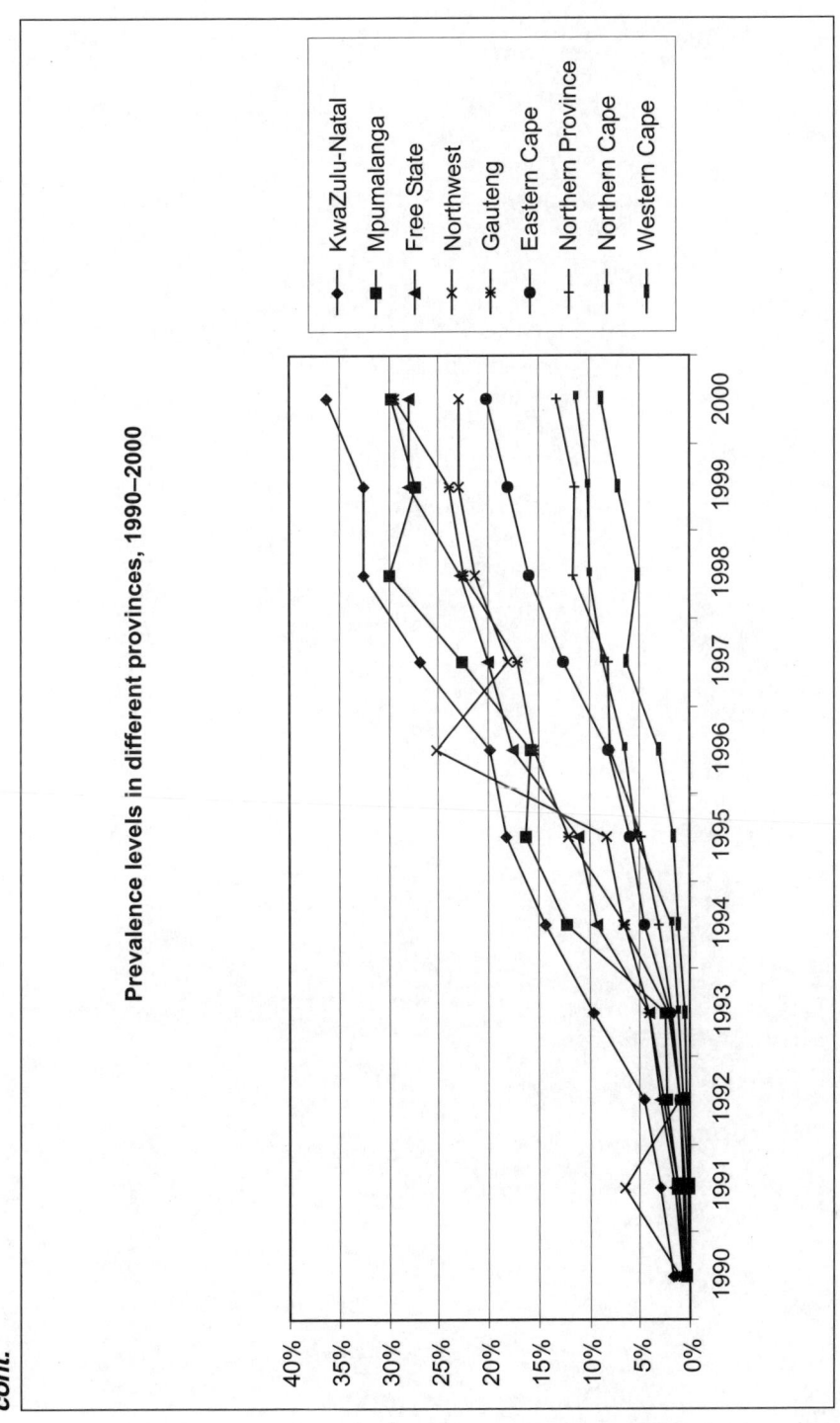

**Prevalence levels in different provinces, 1990–2000**

CHAPTER 3

# Health

*Sonja Giese*

## Introduction

This chapter examines the impact of the HIV/AIDS epidemic on the health of children in South Africa. Perhaps the most startling evidence of this impact is the effect that the AIDS epidemic is expected to have on child health indicators, morbidity and mortality of women and young adults, and the number of children who will be orphaned. These trends as outlined in the previous chapter suggest that there will be a reversal in the gains achieved in improving child health indicators. Increased morbidity and mortality in young adults reduces the pool of caregivers and breadwinners, leaving an increasing number of children in conditions of poverty and neglect. The orphan epidemic is a crisis in its own right with over one million orphans expected within the next ten years. AIDS orphans are arguably the most vulnerable children in our society, struggling not only to survive, but to do so within the context of open discrimination.

The health, developmental and psycho-social impacts of HIV/AIDS on three particularly vulnerable groups of children are discussed in detail in this chapter, namely those living in households where a parent or caregiver is HIV-positive, children who are HIV-positive and those children who are AIDS orphans. Specific reference is made to the impact of HIV on childhood nutritional status. The link between HIV and nutrition is explored at two levels, the first being the destructive cycle of HIV disease progression and malnutrition in HIV-infected children. The second is the impact of HIV on caregiving practices and household food security, which leads to malnutrition in HIV-affected children.

The chapter then looks at the impact of HIV/AIDS on health services for children. In order to accurately determine this impact, reliable data is needed on the numbers of children who will be accessing these services. Of particular concern is the complete absence of data in some areas (such as the number of children who acquire HIV as a result of sexual abuse and the number of children living in child-headed households) and the contradictory data available in other areas such as the number of children under the age of 14 years who are HIV-positive.

## The impacts of HIV/AIDS on children's health

The impact of HIV/AIDS on child health will almost certainly be reflected in a reversal of the gains that have been achieved in improving child health indicators over the past ten years.

### Children living in HIV-affected households

By 2011, 56 per cent of the population will live in households where at least one person is HIV-positive or has died of AIDS. The burden of caring for the sick and destitute will have an impact on the 44 per cent of uninfected households (Haarman, 2001).

At the household level, the impact of HIV/AIDS on children is exacerbated by the fact that HIV usually strikes more than one member of an infected household and this usually includes the primary caregiver and/or breadwinner. When a family member has AIDS, the average household income will fall while expenditure increases with the costs of special medical treatment, transport to health facilities, nutritional requirements and ultimately, funeral costs. The financial impact of an AIDS-related death on the average family is greater than the financial impact of any other cause of death (Steinberg et al., 2000).

The financial burden of HIV/AIDS adversely affects the living standards and quality of life of all household members, leading to food insecurity, malnutrition, poor hygiene, loss of opportunity and other factors related to poverty.

With competing priorities for limited resources, children in infected households are often unable to afford school uniforms, school fees and books which are a prerequisite for school attendance. The combined socio-economic consequences of HIV/AIDS on children in infected households is far reaching, with reduced opportunity for growth and development creating a cycle of dependency, vulnerability and abuse.

> Sizwe has no rights. He is a ten year old boy living in one of the richest countries in Africa, under one of the finest constitutions in the world, but he has no rights. Sizwe looks after his dying mother and two sisters in a mud-block house north of Durban. He left school last year when his mother was sent home from hospital to die because her bed was needed by someone who might recover. He can't go back to school

> because there is no money to buy food or pay for school fees. Sizwe sends his sisters off to beg for mealie meal from a neighbour who sometimes helps out. He leaves his mother sleeping while he makes his third trip of the day to fetch water from the standpipe. When he returns his sisters are waiting with a packet containing a cupful of mealie meal. Sizwe makes a fire while the older girl rocks the toddler to stop her from crying. The mother sleeps between bouts of coughing. It is nearly time. Tomorrow he will visit the lady from the burial society to see if he can get help preparing for the funeral.
>
> (Ewing, 2000)

**Caregiving in affected households**
As the traditional primary caregiver of children, the impact of HIV on women in infected households has a direct impact on the children in those households.

More than 35 per cent of households are headed by women, and 60 per cent of these households live in poverty (May et al., 1998). In HIV-infected households, women carry the burden of caring for the sick and dying as well as the responsibility of caring for the children in the household.

Women are also more vulnerable than men to HIV infection for biological, social and economic reasons. For every ten women infected globally, eight are African women in sub-Saharan Africa and for every one new male infection, two women are infected (Sozi, 2001). Anything that threatens the health of a caregiver, impacts on the health and wellbeing of the child. Uninfected children born to infected mothers have a 2.4–3.6 times greater chance of dying than children born to uninfected mothers (Department of Welfare, 2000a). Also, there is a direct relationship between the severity of maternal disease and the risk of the child acquiring opportunistic infections and dying early in life (Mpanju-Shumbusho, 2001).

**Child health and wellbeing in affected households**
Poor health and increased rates of stunting among children living in HIV-infected families, is common. This is believed to be a consequence of HIV disease itself (in the case of mother to child transmission (MTCT)), increased exposure to opportunistic infections, disease related poverty and psycho-social factors which impact on caregiving practices and child wellbeing (Piwoz and Preble, 2000). Children living in households with HIV-infected persons are more exposed to opportunistic infections, such as tuberculosis (TB) and pneumonia. With caregivers sporadically sick or absent, the child is less likely to get the medical attention s/he needs and more likely to have repeat infections.

Food security in HIV-infected households is affected by reduced household income and increased expenditure on healthcare which leaves less money available to purchase appropriate food. Preparation of food is also affected by compromised caregiving. The child may also be unable or unwilling to eat due to a range of physical, emotional and psycho-social factors which play a role in appetite suppression.

Two other features of HIV-infected households which impact on the health and welfare of children are those of domestic violence and abandonment. Domestic violence is common among HIV-infected families and has become one of the major stumbling blocks to disclosure among married women (Williams 2001). The fear of disclosure makes it difficult for women to make informed decisions on choices such as breastfeeding, family planning and planning for the future of her existing children without raising suspicion about her HIV status. She is therefore forced into continued child bearing and breastfeeding which may significantly compromise the health of her children. The fear of disclosure also means that women are reluctant to accept the assistance of home-based caregivers who may have been able to assist with the care of the children in the infected household.

Abandonment may happen at two levels. The first is the abandonment of the family by a caregiver/breadwinner. It is commonplace to hear of women whose partners or husbands abandoned them when they disclosed their HIV status to their partner. The second is the abandonment of the child. Over the past three years, there has been reported a 67 per cent increase in the number of children abandoned (South African National Council for Child and Family Welfare, 1999). This is corroborated by reports of an increase in the numbers of children being abandoned in hospital wards across the country. Many of these cases could have been prevented if effective social security measures were in place to support desperate families affected by HIV/AIDS.

Children living in an infected household face the double burden of prejudice related to HIV and prejudice related to poverty. They are forced to endure teasing and are marginalised by their peers and other members of their community. Many of these children will be left without a concerned caregiver once their parent dies and the oldest child's role in the family may change. Assuming the role of caregiver makes the girl child particularly vulnerable to sexual abuse by adult men in the household and in turn, vulnerable to HIV infection.

**Children orphaned by HIV/AIDS**
There are already approximately 300 000 maternal AIDS orphans, yet the orphan epidemic is still in its infancy, and over the next few years is expected to grow to devastating proportions. In most parts of the industrialised world,

no more than one per cent of the child population is orphaned. In developing countries this figure was around 2.5 per cent before the HIV/AIDS epidemic (Loening-Voysey and Wilson, 2001). If one combines all other causes of maternal death with the HIV/AIDS epidemic, 11 per cent of children under the age of 15 years are orphans and this figure is expected to dramatically rise by 2010. By 2015, AIDS orphans will constitute between nine and 12 per cent of South Africa's total population.

The 1997 White Paper on Social Development outlined a shift in emphasis towards developmental social welfare that fosters independence and empowers communities. In line with this, the extended family and other community-based models of care are the preferred options for placement of children who have been orphaned. However, as a result of the HIV/AIDS epidemic, huge numbers of children are being orphaned and the existing pool of community-based support is becoming saturated. Evidence of this can be seen in the large and increasing numbers of child- and sibling-headed households.

**Care and support of orphans**
In the developing world, societies traditionally absorb orphans into the extended family or community. There are six existing approaches to care of orphans (Loening-Voysey and Wilson, 2001):

1. informal/non-statutory fostering (with little support from the community or government);
2. community-based support structures/family foster care with community support (informal fostering with community support);
3. home-based care and support;
4. unregistered/non-statutory residential care;
5. statutory foster care;
6. statutory residential care.

The approach being encouraged by government favours approaches two and three. As a result of the HIV/AIDS epidemic, huge numbers of children are being orphaned and traditional support structures like approach six is largely saturated. Government has chosen to move away from residential care as an option and wishes to rely upon the extended family or other members in communities to care for orphans. The decision to scale up family and community support mechanisms and scale down statutory foster and residential care ties in with the international research findings. It also flows naturally from the shift of the Department of Social Development (Welfare) from a residential care approach to a developmental approach in the delivery of services. It has been found that the extended family and kinship networks are able to provide better quality services to orphans than residential-based models of care

(Loening-Voysey and Wilson, 2001). These types of care can be delivered at a lower cost and that the caregiving efforts of extended families and kinship networks need to be supported (Desmond and Gow, 2001). However, the stigma associated with AIDS is such that children orphaned by HIV/AIDS are at risk of being turned away by extended families fearful of the consequences of caring for them.

> 'Before this tragedy struck my family, I had a lot of friends and we lived in close community with our neighbours. But after my parents died, and it became known that AIDS had killed them, they all started to drift away. Today we can't even ask our neighbours for a pinch of salt because, when we approach them, they demand to know what we want and don't allow us to enter their yard' – 18 year old Avhapfani, Northern Province.
>
> *Sunday Times*, 11 June 2000

Degrees of vulnerability exist within the broad group of children defined as orphans, with the most vulnerable orphans being those living on the streets or in child-headed households. For those children for whom caregivers are found, groups of siblings are often split between households. It is quite common for orphans to be cared for by grandparents or great grandparents who die while the child is still young. Many children therefore experience a string of multiple caregivers before they finally reach the age of independence. Older orphans are frequently exploited by their caregivers. They may be forced to leave school and perform chores in and around the house, or they may be expected to seek employment to subsidise the household income.

If suitable caregivers are not available, some children may become responsible for the care of younger siblings, living in child-headed households. The problem of child-headed households is poorly understood and data on the number of children currently living in child-headed households is scant (Statistics South Africa, 2001). While there have been increases in the number of children living in households without parental supervision, home-based caregivers report that older siblings (over the age of 18 years) are fulfilling the role of caregiver, having left school early to provide for the needs of younger siblings. Children living in child-headed households typically live in conditions of poverty, without adequate adult supervision and suffer from stunting and hunger. These children have reduced opportunities for education, limited access to health and welfare services and no access to social security. For many, they assume the role of caregiver at a very young age. Older children may be exploited and forced into child labour, prostitution or early marriage. Some leave home to supplement the household income through begging in city centres, thereby increasing the numbers of street children.

Many child-headed households face eviction from their homes, either through property grabbing by greedy relatives or because they are unable to sustain mortgage agreements and are too young to access a housing subsidy.

> 'Shouldering a burden weightier than his 15 years, Langanani Mugodo picks up a cast-iron pot and, seemingly without a second thought, breaks centuries of Venda tradition. He walks outside into the sun-baked centre of the kraal, squats on the earth near a hollow and, gathering his domestic tools about him, lights the cooking fire. This is exclusively women's work and Langanani has trespassed, breaking the gender barriers which still define social roles in this far flung rural part of the Northern Province. After his parents died of AIDS, as the eldest son, Langanani became head of the household and responsible for feeding his 5 siblings. 'After my mother died when I was 13, I had to stop going to school and instead had to learn how to cook meals for my brother and sisters. I also sweep the home and fetch water, all the things which women usually do. But there was no one there to help us. At first my school friends mocked me because I was doing girls' work. But now I think they understand I have no choice'.
> 
> *Marie Claire*, November 2000

## Impact on child health and wellbeing

Children who have been orphaned are more likely than their peers to be malnourished, sick, abused and sexually exploited. They are at greater risk of dying from preventable diseases and are less likely than other children to be fully immunised. This has implications for all children. As immunisation coverage decreases, the herd immunity declines and all children become more susceptible to common childhood illnesses which in the case of HIV-infected children, can be fatal.

With limited resources and inadequate adult supervision, orphans are more likely than their peers to drop out of school, leaving them with fewer opportunities for growth and development. They are also denied the benefit of the monitoring and support of teachers and peers and the nutritional support offered through the primary school nutrition programme which targets poor children at schools.

> 17 year old Nyawo cares for her 3 younger siblings. The family fails to qualify for government child support grants as all the children are over the age of 7 years and Nyawo is too young to access a foster grant. 'I am very worried because I can't understand why, being so young, I have to carry the burden of elders. If there is no food at home, these children look to me to do something.' The plea from Nyawo and other orphans is for the government to feed and clothe them and pay their school fees.
>
> *Cape Times*, 17 April 2001

While these issues affect children orphaned for any reason, as a result of the stigma and discrimination surrounding AIDS and the devastating socio-economic consequences of the virus, children orphaned by HIV/AIDS are at greater risk than other orphans (UNAIDS, 2000).

The psychological impact on the child of witnessing the suffering and death of a parent is extreme. For many children this is exacerbated by the fear and insecurity of not knowing who will care for and support them after their parents' death. Many households with terminally ill AIDS patients survive on the Adult Disability Grant or a pension which is stopped once the adult recipient dies. AIDS orphans often face the additional burden of not being able to grieve openly for a deceased loved one because of the stigma associated with an AIDS-related death. The long term effects of this is likely to plague the country for many years to come, with desperate and disillusioned youth turning to anti-social and risk taking behaviour and crime.

One of the most severe and lasting consequences of parental death is childhood malnutrition (Piwoz and Preble, 2000). The impact of HIV on the nutritional status of a child is felt long before the parent's death and, if ongoing and severe, can have a long-term impact on the development of the child. Many of these children will also be infected with HIV and for most of them, access to essential drugs and social security will be limited.

**Children infected with HIV**
HIV/AIDS attacks not only the most productive members of society but also the most vulnerable. Children infected with HIV live in affected households and for many of these children, one or more of their parents will also be HIV-positive. All the stresses and socio-economic consequences of living in an HIV-infected household therefore apply to these children in addition to the burden of HIV infection.

## HIV transmission in children

The majority of HIV-infected children under the age of 13 years acquire HIV from their infected mothers during pregnancy, at the time of delivery, or after birth through breastfeeding. Over 105 000 babies were born HIV-positive in 2000 (Department of Health, 2000). Sixty per cent of these children will not live beyond their 5th birthday. Forty per cent of them will survive, and the majority of these children will join the 60–70 per cent of children who live in conditions of extreme poverty (Haarmann, 2001). These children will be vulnerable to abuse, neglect and exploitation and will almost certainly have reduced opportunities and limited access to basic services.

Fifteen to 18 year olds fall within the age category most vulnerable to HIV infection through sexual contact. Within this group, girls are particularly vulnerable to infection. Physiological, cultural and social factors contribute to the vulnerability of the girl child and girls between the ages of 5 and 14 years are more than eight times more likely to be infected through sexual abuse than their male counterparts (Shell, 2000). In sub-Saharan Africa, the rate of HIV infection in teenage girls is five times higher than the rate of infection in teenage boys (Mpanju-Shumbusho, 2001).

The extent to which sexual abuse contributes to HIV infection in children is not known. Models (such as the ASSA2000 model), used to calculate the number of people infected, are based on the assumption that mother to child transmission is 100 per cent accountable for infections in children under the age of 14 years. This is despite the fact that there has been a marked increase in the numbers of children who are sexually abused over the last ten years. At Edendale hospital, for example, two cases of child sexual abuse were reported in 1989. By 1996 the number of reported cases rose to 306. While it is acknowledged that this increase could be a result of increased awareness or improved services for children, HIV could be playing a significant role in this upward spiral. One way in which HIV could be contributing is that, with the high rates of infection, young children are seen as safe partners. The myth that sex with a virgin cures AIDS is another potential contributing factor (McKerrow, 1997). A study conducted at a child abuse centre in a tertiary hospital in KwaZulu-Natal found that, taking into account the likely rate of transmission in children and the HIV prevalence in the area, a disproportionate number of children who were raped acquired HIV. This supports the hypothesis that virgins (children) are the victims of targeted rape by HIV-positive adults (McKerrow, 1997).

There are also no accurate figures on the number of children infected through unsafe health practices (such as unscreened blood products or the use of contaminated medical instruments) and traditional practices such as scarification and circumcision.

Certain groups of children are particularly vulnerable to HIV infection. These include child sex workers, street children, children in detention, children using intravenous drugs (or other substances which lead to risk taking behaviour) and orphans (Sozi, 2001).

### HIV disease progression in children

Disease progression among HIV-positive children in Africa is relatively rapid with a small proportion of children remaining asymptomatic for longer periods (slow progressors). Disease progression may be exacerbated in the South African setting by increased exposure to infections and high rates of malnutrition. Approximately one-third of infants infected with HIV through MTCT die before their 1st birthday and two-thirds die by their 5th birthday (Piwoz and Preble, 2000).

The most common features of clinical paediatric HIV are pulmonary infections (such as pneumonia and TB), persistent diarrhoea, growth failure, swollen lymph nodes, chronic cough and fever. These features of paediatric HIV are also common in non-HIV-infected children with the major difference being that in HIV-infected children these tend to be more severe and frequent (Luo and Coulter, 2001). Low birth weight in HIV-infected newborns also contributes to increased perinatal mortality and morbidity.

HIV disease progression in children acquiring HIV through MTCT can be divided into two main categories:

1. Rapid progressors – infants who become symptomatic and very sick within a few months of birth and usually die by the age of 2 years.
2. Slow progressors – children who remain asymptomatic or present with less severe symptoms during the first two years. These children generally survive to older childhood.

Poorer prognoses are associated with higher viral load, increased virulence of the virus, poor nutritional status of the child, concurrent infections (such as measles or TB) and lower economic status. In most settings in sub-Saharan Africa, the medication available for an HIV-positive child is even less than that available for an adult and most facilities are not geared to care for the chronically sick adolescent (Sozi, 2001).

## *Understanding the relationship between HIV and nutrition*

Malnutrition has been an endemic problem in Africa for decades and now research suggests that it is intricately linked with HIV (Piwoz and Preble, 2000). Malnutrition is one of the biggest contributors to childhood morbidity and mortality (Child Health Policy Institute, 1999). The recent national food consumption survey found that, in children aged under ten years, one in five are stunted and one in ten are underweight (Department of Welfare, 2000b).

The impact of HIV/AIDS on childhood malnutrition can be observed at many levels. HIV infection in children compromises their nutritional status and with poor nutritional status, disease progression is hastened. This creates a vicious cycle that undermines the health of the infected child. In HIV-negative children living in HIV-infected households the impact of HIV on nutrition is seen in reduced food security and compromised caregiving.

Another way in which HIV/AIDS may be impacting on childhood nutritional status is through the controversy surrounding breastfeeding. The link between HIV transmission and breastfeeding has placed policymakers and healthcare workers in a difficult predicament. It has been shown that HIV can be transmitted through breast milk but often mothers do not have access to a clean water supply to make up formula. The infant may, therefore, be at greater risk of dying from diarrhoeal disease as a result of unsafe water than from contracting HIV through breast milk. In the absence of clear guidelines, the controversy surrounding this issue could impact on breastfeeding practices and therefore on childhood nutrition.

**The vicious cycle of HIV infection and malnutrition**
Children admitted to hospitals with HIV related illnesses commonly present with severe malnutrition (Cotton et al., 1998). The changes in the immune system functioning due to HIV is very similar to changes in the immune system as a result of malnutrition and poor nutritional status can therefore hasten disease progression.

HIV infection impacts on the nutritional status of infected children through a variety of direct and indirect means (Piwoz and Preble, 2000):

- Reductions in dietary intake is common in children who are infected/affected by HIV/AIDS. HIV infection in a family is typically associated with reduced household income and therefore reduced food availability. Furthermore caregivers may themselves be sick and unable to provide the child with a healthy meal. The child may be unable or unwilling to consume food due to depression, fatigue or other psycho-social factors that play a role in appetite suppression. Sores in the mouth and throat are common in HIV-positive children and make chewing and swallowing food painful. If the child is on medication, side effects from the medication may contribute to reduced dietary intake, e.g. by making the child nauseous (Piwoz, 2001).
- Nutrient malabsorption in children is predominantly a result of frequent and persistent diarrhoea. Fat malabsorption in children is common at all stages

of HIV infection and makes it difficult for the child's body to absorb and utilise important fat-soluble vitamins such as Vitamins A and E.
- Changes in the body's metabolism occur during HIV infection. This is a result of severe reductions in food intake (as described above) as well as the immune system's response which triggers an increased utilisation and excretion of micronutrients.

The body's immune response is intricately linked to the body's nutritional status and as the body tries to fight off the HIV, a vicious cycle develops as Figure 3.1 shows.

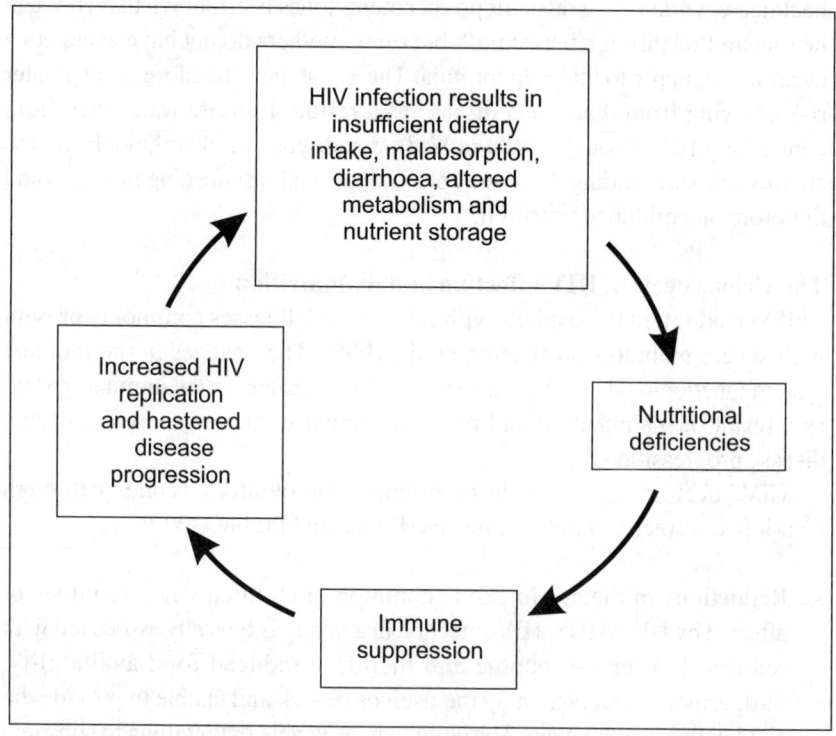

Source: Semba and Tang (1999)

**Figure 3.1 The vicious cycle of micronutrient deficiencies and human immunodeficiency virus (HIV) pathogenesis.**

## Food security and caregiving practices

The impact of HIV/AIDS on the country's economy and on health and welfare services means that human, economic, material and institutional resources are stretched. This impacts on individual households in areas such as hygiene, sanitation, health and food security.

In addition to this, HIV/AIDS attacks caregivers and breadwinners within the household, reducing the resources available to purchase food and the caregiver's ability to provide the child with a nutritionally balanced diet.

At various levels therefore, HIV/AIDS impacts on the nutritional status of children living in HIV-infected households, leaving them more susceptible to malnutrition, growth faltering, disease and micronutrient deficiency related ailments.

Figure 3.2 below illustrates the link between broader household and societal issues and malnutrition in children.

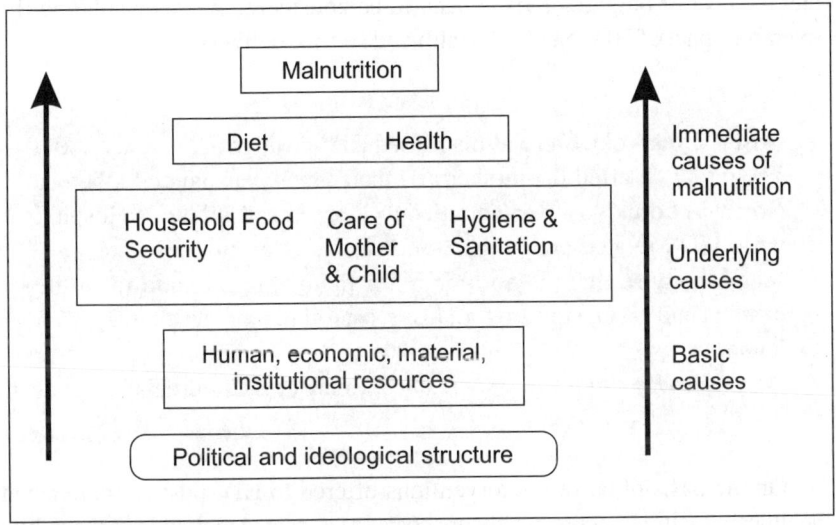

Source: Piwoz (2001)

Figure 3.2  Causes of malnutrition in children.

## The impact of HIV on health services for children

Studies of paediatric admissions in hospitals have shown a marked increase in HIV-related admissions (Zwi et al., 1999). HIV-positive children spend an estimated 3.4 times longer in hospital and require multiple admissions (Cotton et al., 1998). In 1997 and 1998, 20 per cent of paediatric admissions at Chris Hani Baragwanath Hospital were HIV related (Zwi et al., 1999). In 1999 over half of the admissions to King Edward VIII Hospital in Durban were HIV related (Colvin and Kleinschmidt, 2000). Increases in paediatric admissions in general over the past few years are significant and entirely attributable to

HIV/AIDS (Mpanju-Shumbusho, 2001). In areas of the country with very high rates of infection, up to 75 per cent of beds in the children's wards are occupied by children with AIDS-related conditions (Barrett et al., 1999). As a result of the increased burden on health services, children suffering from conditions other than HIV will have to wait longer for access to a hospital bed and it can expected that there will be an increase in mortality among HIV-negative patients due to delayed treatment. As the epidemic progresses and more HIV-positive people develop AIDS, the impact on the health sector will grow exponentially.

The most obvious costs in caring for HIV-positive children are those incurred by the healthcare facility itself, but additional costs such as the cost to the parents for transport to and from hospital, reduced household income and the cost of outpatient visits need to be considered when calculating the overall impact of HIV on child health and service delivery.

> Nosi is 2 years old. She was diagnosed HIV-positive in February 2001. The father deserted the mother and their three-year-old child, before Nosi was born. Nosi was admitted to Red Cross Children's Hospital with AIDS-related symptoms a month ago. Her mother's visits are scarce because there is no money for the bus fare to and from the hospital and no-one to care for Nosi's sister if her mother is away from home.
>
> *Personal Correspondence*, Red Cross Children's Hospital

On the basis of current interventions offered to HIV-positive patients at healthcare facilities, acute healthcare costs are expected to double in the public sector by 2010. The estimated cost per year of treating an HIV-positive individual with the interventions currently available at public sector healthcare facilities is R17 000 (stage 4 of disease), R6 200 (stage 3) and R1 300 (stage 1 and 2) (Steinberg et al., 2000). Government will be pressurised into increasing its expenditure on health services and the specific share of the budget allocated to the care of HIV-infected individuals. At the same time, rationing of services will have to occur as projected expenditure requirements are not sustainable.

Rationing of services for HIV-positive children in healthcare facilities has already begun with HIV-positive children being denied access to intensive care units in some provinces (Schneider and Russel, 2000). Many HIV-positive children are also diagnosed early as rapid progressors and denied access to medication on the assumption that the medication will do little to extend their life. In a further attempt to deal with the epidemic, patients are being referred away from health facilities to more community-based programmes such as home-based care. Home-based models of care have been found to be very effective in reducing rate of hospitalisation and length of stay in hospital, reducing the impact of HIV/AIDS on primary healthcare services, reducing the costs and providing support for the family and increasing compliance to treatment regimes (Johnson et al., 2001). It is not surprising then that this is being promoted by policymakers, but the existing health system lacks the infrastructure and resources to provide the necessary training and support to home-based carers (Whiteside, 2000).

Healthcare workers face difficult decisions as hospitals move towards providing palliative care for children with AIDS. All of these factors are likely to have an impact on the psychological wellbeing of service providers and increase rates of burnout and incidence of job-related stress.

The growing demand on healthcare services is exacerbated by an escalating TB epidemic, developing in the shadows of HIV. Currently, about half of all TB cases are thought to be attributable to HIV (Allen et al., 2000). As HIV weakens the immune system, it makes people more vulnerable to opportunistic infections and to developing active TB. With a greater number of HIV-positive people developing TB, HIV-positive and HIV-negative children will be exposed to a greater number of potential sources of TB infection (Schaaf et al., 2000). The World Bank estimates that 25 per cent of TB-related deaths in HIV-negative people in the coming years will be a direct result of the HIV/AIDS epidemic (UNAIDS, 2000). In the Western Cape, the number of TB cases continue to increase, mainly due to HIV/AIDS and each new case of TB represents a further drain on the health system (Western Cape Department of Health, 2001).

The impact of HIV/AIDS on the health sector will also be felt through HIV-related illness and death of healthcare workers. While increasing the demand on the healthcare system, HIV simultaneously reduces the system's capacity to cope with the epidemic by killing healthcare workers, the majority of whom are women. Rising rates of HIV infection among healthcare workers will lead to increased absenteeism, reduced productivity and greater spending on treatment, death benefits, staff recruitment and training of new personnel. The burden of the HIV/AIDS epidemic will divert resources from other essential healthcare services and make it difficult to implement and maintain other key primary healthcare programmes.

## *Conclusion*
HIV/AIDS impacts on children to different degrees and at different levels. For children living in HIV-infected households, children orphaned by HIV/AIDS

and children who are HIV-positive, their basic rights to food, housing and healthcare are violated to the extent that their survival is threatened. The impact of HIV/AIDS on children and families is compounded by the fact that most infected families already live in poverty-stricken communities with limited access to basic services and poor infrastructure.

In an effort to mitigate the impact of HIV/AIDS on child survival, crisis management has taken over. As a result, there is a risk of ignoring the less urgent but no less severe impact of HIV/AIDS on the child's psycho-social wellbeing, intellectual development, education, and right to participate in an engaging society and be protected from abuse and discrimination.

Health and social development services are not equipped to deal with the onslaught of the AIDS epidemic and community-based structures need support, monitoring and financial resources.

HIV/AIDS demands a co-ordinated and holistic response from government, the private sector, non-governmental organisations and civil society. 2002 is at a turning point in the history of South Africa. The actions or apathy in tackling the epidemic will determine the future growth and development of the country.

## References

Allen, D., N. Simelela and L. Makubalo. 2000. 'Epidemiology of HIV/AIDS in South Africa'. *Southern African Journal of HIV Medicine* 1: 9–11.

Barrett, C., N. McKerrow and A. Strode. 1999. 'Consultative Paper on Children Living with HIV/AIDS'. Unpublished paper prepared for the South African Law Commission, Pretoria.

Bradshaw, D., K. Masiteng and N. Nannan. 2001. 'Health Status and Determinants'. In *South African Health Review 2000*, A. Ntuli, N. Crisp, E. Clarke and P. Barron (eds). Durban: Health Systems Trust.

Child Health Policy Institute. 1999. *Children in South Africa: Their Right to Health*. Cape Town: University of Cape Town.

Child Health Unit. 1998. *HIV/AIDS and the Family: A Clinical Guide*. Cape Town: University of Cape Town.

Clacherty and Associates 2001. 'The Experiences and Concerns of Children and Youth Affected by HIV/AIDS'. Report on participatory workshops for Soul Buddyz 2, Johannesburg, April.

Colvin, M. and I. Kleinschmidt. 2000. 'The Impact of HIV/AIDS on Medical Wards of a Tertiary Hospital in KwaZulu-Natal'. *Southern African Journal of HIV Medicine* 1: 14–17.

Cotton, M., H. Schaaf, E. Willemsen, M. van Veenendal, A. van Rensburg and E. van Rensburg. 1998. 'The Burden of Mother-to-Child Transmission of HIV-

1 Disease in a Low Prevalence Region: A Five year Study of Hospitalised Children'. *South African Journal of Epidemiology and Infection* 13(2): 46–49.

Coutsoudis, A. 2000. 'Method of Feeding and Transmission of HIV-1 from Mothers to Children by 15 months of Age: Prospective Cohort Study from Durban'. Paper presented at 13th International AIDS conference, Durban.

Department of Health 2000. *National HIV and Syphilis Sero-Prevalence Survey of Women Attending Public Antenatal Clinics in South Africa*. Pretoria.

Department of Welfare 2000a. *National Strategic Framework for Children Infected and Affected by HIV/AIDS*. Pretoria.

Department of Welfare 2000b. *National Food Consumption Survey in Children Aged 1–9 Years: South Africa*. Pretoria.

Department of Welfare 2001. *National Workshop on Social Security for Children in South Africa*. March. Pretoria.

Department of Welfare and Population Development. 1997. *White Paper for Social Welfare*. Pretoria.

Desmond, C. and J. Gow. 2001. *The Cost Effectiveness of Six Models of Care for Orphan and Vulnerable Children in South Africa*. Pretoria: UNICEF.

Dray-Spira, R., P. Lepage and F. Dabis. 2000. 'Prevention of Infectious Complications of Paediatric HIV Infection in Africa'. *AIDS* 14: 1091–1099.

Ewing, D. 2000. 'Children and AIDS: Prevention Means Access to Treatment Now'. *Children First* 4(32): 4.

Free State Department of Health 2001. 'Health budget hearings presentation'. April. Reported in Health-e. (accessed March 2002). www.health-e.org.za/view.php3?id

Gauteng Department of Health 2001. 'Health budget hearings presentation'. April. Reported in Health-e. (accessed March 2002). www.health-e.org.za/view.php3?id

Giese, S. and G. Hussey. 2002. *A Rapid Appraisal of Primary Level Health Care Services for HIV Positive Children at Public Sector Clinics in South Africa*. Cape Town: Children's Institute and Child Health Unit, University of Cape Town.

Giese, S., P. Proudlock and H. Meintjes. 2002. *Draft Report on the National Children's Forum on HIV/AIDS*. Cape Town: Children's Institute, University of Cape Town.

Haarmann, C. 2001. *Social Assistance in South Africa: Its Potential Impact on Poverty*. PhD thesis, University of the Western Cape, Cape Town.

Johnson, L. and R. Dorrington. 2001. *The Impact of AIDS on Orphanhood in South Africa: A Quantitative Analysis*. Cape Town: Centre for Actuarial Science, University of Cape Town.

Johnson, S., P. Modiba, D. Monnakgotla, D. Muirhead and H. Schneider. 2001. *Home-Based Care for People with HIV/AIDS in South Africa*. Johannesburg: Centre for Health Policy, Department of Community Health, University of the Witwatersrand.

Lorey, M. 1999. Foreword. *AIDS Orphan Alert*. Lutry, Switzerland: Association Francois – Xavier Bagnoud.

Loening-Voysey, H. and T. Wilson. 2001. *Approaches to Caring for Children Orphaned by AIDS and other Vulnerable Children: Essential Elements for a Quality Service*. Pretoria: UNICEF.

Luo, C. and B. Coulter. 2001. 'Diagnosis of Paediatric HIV Infection in Africa'. Paper presented at National Institute of Health Gaborone conference, March.

May, J., D. Budlender, R. Mokate, C. Rogerson, A. Stavrou and N. Wilkins. 1998. *Poverty and Inequality: Report Prepared for the Office of the Executive Deputy President and the Inter-Ministerial Committee for Poverty and Inequality*. Durban: Praxis Publishing.

McKerrow, N. 1997. 'Childhood Sexual Abuse and HIV/AIDS'. Paper presented at the South African Society for Prevention of Child Abuse and Neglect National Conference, Durban.

Motala, S. 2001. 'Children in South Africa: A Contextual Analysis'. Paper presented at National Workshop on Social Security for Children in South Africa, March.

Mpanju-Shumbusho, W. 2001. 'A Historic Overview of the Progression of HIV/AIDS Epidemic in Sub-Saharan Africa and its Impact on Women and Children'. Paper presented at the National Institute of Health Gaborone conference, March.

Musoke, P. 2001. 'Opportunistic Infections and Complications of HIV Infected African Children'. Paper presented at National Institute of Health Gaborone conference, March.

Nduati, R. 2001.'Research for HIV/AIDS Care in Women and Children'. Paper presented at the National Institute of Health Gaborone conference, March.

Piwoz, E. and E. Preble. 2000. *HIV/AIDS and Nutrition: A Review of the Literature and Recommendations for Nutritional Care and Support in Sub-Saharan Africa*. Washington: Academy for Educational Development.

Piwoz, E. 2001. 'Diet, Nutrition and HIV/AIDS: What is the Connection?' Paper presented at the National Institute of Health Gaborone conference, March.

The Presidency. 1999. *President's Report on the State of the Nation's Children*. Pretoria.

Schaaf, H., M. Cotton, G. de Villiers and P. Donald. 2000. 'Clinical Insights into the Interaction of Childhood Tuberculosis and HIV in the Western Cape'. *Southern African Journal of HIV Medicine* 1: 33–35.

Schneider, H. and M. Russell. 2000. *A Rapid Appraisal of Community-Based HIV/AIDS Care and Support in South Africa*. Johannesburg: Centre for Health Policy, Department of Community Health, University of the Witwatersrand.

Semba, R. and A. Tang. 1999. 'Micronutrients and the Pathogenesis of Human Immunodeficiency Virus Infection'. *British Journal of Nutrition* 81(3): 181–189.

Shell, R. 2000. 'AIDS in the Poorest Province of South Africa, 1976 to 2001'. Working Paper 8. DEMSA Annual Conference, Port Elizabeth, October.

Smart, R. 1999. *Children Living with HIV/AIDS in South Africa: A Rapid Appraisal*. Johannesburg: Save the Children.

Smith, C. 2000. *Mail and Guardian*, 21–27 July.

South African Law Commission 1998. *The Review of the Child Care Act*. Issue Paper 13. Pretoria.

South African Law Commission. 2000. *Submission to the Committee of Inquiry into a Comprehensive Social Security System*. October. Pretoria.

South African National Council for Child and Family Welfare. 1999. *Annual Report*. Johannesburg.

Sozi, S. 2001. 'The Scope of the Problem of Providing Care to Women and Children Affected by HIV/AIDS in Sub Saharan Africa and the Response to Date'. Paper presented at the National Institute of Health Gaborone conference, March.

Statistics South Africa. 2001. 'Children's Statistical Newsletter 8', January/February. (accessed March 2002).
www.statssa.gov.za

Steinberg, M., A. Kinghorn, N. Soderlund, G. Schierhout and S. Conway. 2000. HIV/AIDS: Facts Figures and the Future. In *South African Health Review 2000*, A. Ntuli, N. Crisp, E. Clarke and P. Barron (eds). Durban: Health Systems Trust.

Strachan, K. and E. Clarke. 2000. *Everybody's Business: The Enlightening Truth About AIDS*. Cape Town: Metropolitan Group.

UNAIDS. 1998. *Report on the Global HIV/AIDS epidemic: June 1998*. Geneva: United Nations.

UNAIDS. 2000. *Report on the Global HIV/AIDS epidemic: June 2000*. Geneva: United Nations.

Western Cape Department of Health. 2001. 'Health budget hearings presentation'. April. Reported in Health-e. (accessed March 2002).
www.health-e.org.za/view.php3?id

Williams, E. 2001. 'Understanding Social and Behavioural Factors in African Settings that Impact on HIV Treatment, Care and Management of Women and Children'. Paper presented at National Institute of Health Gaborone conference, March.

Zwi, K., J. Pettifor and N. Soderlund. 1999. 'Paediatric Hospital Admissions at a South African Urban Regional Hospital: The Impact of HIV, 1992–1997'. *Annals of Tropical Paediatrics* 19: 135–142.

CHAPTER 4

# Welfare

*Deborah Ewing*

## *Introduction*

This chapter presents a critical discussion of the impact on HIV/AIDS on child welfare and associated levels of child poverty in South Africa. It draws on official data, independent studies, reports from non-govermental organisations (NGOs) and AIDS support groups, case studies and interviews with adults and children affected by AIDS. The discussion refers to the impact of HIV/AIDS upon all children, including:

- children infected with HIV/AIDS;
- children orphaned by HIV/AIDS (fostered, child-headed households, children on the streets);
- children in families with a member living with HIV/AIDS;
- children in families caring for a child orphaned by HIV/AIDS.

While it looks at impacts specifically upon children, not just as members of impoverished households, it also refers to several inter-generational impacts:

- diagnosis, sickness and death of adult carers (the 15–49 age-group being most likely to be infected);
- increased dependency ratio as a result of the declining proportion of economically active adults in the population;
- demand for older people to become caregivers for the second time around;
- impact on tomorrow's adults as potential parents, educators, and leaders whose ability to be healthy, happy and productive members of society is being severely curtailed.

## Background and overview of data and literature

While a broad, qualitative definition of poverty is used by the National Programme of Action for Children (NPA), in line with the Convention on the Rights of the Child (CRC), and while the importance of the qualitative aspects of poverty (vulnerability, lack of decision-making power) is widely accepted in policy and research circles, most available data continues to focus on income indicators of poverty.

Most recent estimates of the child poverty rate vary between 60 per cent (May et al., 1998) and 72 per cent (Haarmann, 1999). These estimates are based on income poverty lines and only the Haarmann study looks at household spending per child as opposed to household income. Such figures provide a baseline for looking at broad trends but not for assessing children's quality of life.

There is a critical lack of data both on child poverty (trends and causal factors) and on children infected or affected by HIV. The State of the Nation's Children 2000 report, commissioned in 1999 by the Office of the President from Statistics South Africa, provides an analysis of the extent and nature of child poverty, which includes a chapter on HIV/AIDS but this is still based largely on the 1996 Census data. The report aims to establish a baseline and highlights the critical lack of data related to the impact of HIV/AIDS, and other impoverishing factors on children.

National and provincial statistical data do not yet incorporate current data on HIV/AIDS. The wealth of data that is being compiled on the current situation regarding HIV/AIDS cannot be easily correlated with key indicators.

The research conducted for the interim National HIV/AIDS Care and Support Task Team provides an up-to-date analysis of the situation of children affected by HIV/AIDS from a rights perspective (Smart, 1999). This was the only research that could be sourced that compiles such a composite national picture, centred on project studies in five provinces, that identifies the needs, responses and gaps in support for children and their families and communities.

It is difficult to disaggregate the impact of HIV/AIDS from other factors in poverty. The bulk of research that considers the links between HIV/AIDS and poverty is concerned with poverty as a co-factor in vulnerability to and spread of HIV/AIDS. The research that looks at the impact of HIV/AIDS on children focuses predominantly on rates of mother to child transmission and the number of orphans. These two issues are usually analysed in terms of scale and potential impact on social spending, not impact on children's right to survival, protection and development.

## Child poverty impacts of HIV/AIDS
### Welfare

Of the 17 million children in South Africa, about 12 million are classified as living in poverty, according to household income indicators. Children account for 25 per cent of those living in poverty. Nine percent of children live in households without either parents or grandparents (ACESS, 2001).

According to the ASSA2000 projections, a total of between five and six million people will probably have died of HIV/AIDS by 2010. 'The number of maternal AIDS orphans (children under the age of 15 whose mothers have died of HIV/AIDS) is expected to rise from some 300 000 currently to around 3 million by 2011'.

The figures show a startling impact on adult mortality. 'Without behavioural change and interventions half of adults can be expected to contract the virus during their life times . . . these effects have the consequence of reducing the life expectancy at birth from over 60 years in the mid-90s to slightly above 40 by 2010.' (UNAIDS, 2000).

There have been many international and national studies looking at the orphan problem. Most concentrate on the issue of scale, the crisis of unmanageability and the imperative of community-based care. Few look at the impact of being orphaned on individual children, or on children and adults in the households into which orphans are absorbed. Some studies have examined the wide range of socio-economic impacts experienced by children in poor, AIDS-affected families (Whiteside, 1998). These point to the all-encompassing breakdown that can begin with the diagnosis or the suspicion of HIV infection in a family.

There is widespread evidence and experience among caregivers, social, health and community workers of the costs (economic, physical, emotional and opportunity) to all members of a poor household affected by AIDS. These costs often outstrip the available resources on every front. This needs to be better documented and given a much higher profile. Otherwise it might appear to policymakers promoting home-based and community-based care as the only affordable option that these costs are, and will continue to be, absorbed.

The Department of Welfare National Strategic Framework for Children Infected and Affected by HIV/AIDS has the two laudable aims of delivering an effective and appropriate care system, and identifying and building on family and community strengths to care for vulnerable children. The Department has recognised the challenge to transform the social security system to address child poverty with particular regard to the impact of AIDS. In the meantime, there is a desperate need to make the existing system deliver to children in households that have exhausted all their strengths.

## Case Study

Cecilia Motaung had not recovered from the shock of losing her eldest daughter Zama before Busi died. She had not found the money for the first funeral before she had to pay for the second. She had been paying into a burial society for five years – thinking it would cover the cost of her own funeral – but when her children became sick she missed some payments and the scheme refused to pay a cent.

When Zama and Busi were well, they supported their mother and their children. Now there are 12 people living in Ma Motaung's two-bedroom house in Clermont, Durban, with no income between them. AIDS has cost this family two daughters, a livelihood, their independence – and with that much of their dignity – and all their prospects of a better life.

'Only God knows how I am coping. I am sick and I am unemployed, and I still have my other children and my grandchildren to look after.' Ma Motaung had thought the family would survive on her disability grant but that was cancelled the month Busi died. Although she has difficulty walking and is dependent on monthly hospital treatment to keep her asthma under control, Ma Motaung was among the many grant recipients who were suddenly informed they were fit to work. A year later she is still waiting for the reinstated grant to be paid – and she owes nearly four times the monthly amount to the funeral director.

Ma Motaung has applied for a foster care grant to help her support her grandchildren. Meanwhile, she has borrowed money to pay their school fees and feeds them on mealie meal given by neighbours. Her diabetic sister has ulcerated feet and can neither walk nor pay taxi fare to the clinic. The sister's youngest child, a severely malnourished seven-year-old, is believed to have suffered a stroke, but several trips to the clinic have yielded nothing but debts. Efforts to secure a child support grant have failed.

The clear reliance upon households and the community is the first line in the care of children and the prevention of child poverty. The experience of many community-based organisations is that this strategy reduces the cost of care to the government, in the short term, but increases the cost to the family and community, in terms of time, energy, emotional and material resources to insupportable levels. Thandanani AIDS orphans community care programme based in Pietermaritzburg warns that the number of orphaned children requiring foster care is growing while community capacity to care for those children without support is shrinking.

Linda Aadnesgaard, of Thandanani, says: 'There still is something left in the sponge in terms of absorption. The spirit is willing but the people are beginning not to cope.' Aadnesgaard says if the government continues to transfer all responsibility for AIDS care to those with the least resources, without adjusting social spending to take account of the burden, the future when the community carers (mostly grandmothers) are burned out or dead is 'too scary to think about'.

By 2010, the number of infected people in the population is likely to peak between seven and eight million, while approximately one million people will be living with AIDS. A total of between five and six million people will probably have died of HIV/AIDS by 2010. The direct and indirect economic impacts of these deaths, combined with existing income inequality and unemployment, are already predicted to be on a scale that cannot be absorbed at national level, let al.one at household level, by children and older people whose financial, material and emotional resources are already exhausted.

Cohen (2000) observed: 'Individuals, families and communities are impoverished by their experience of HIV and AIDS in ways that are typical for long drawn-out and terminal illnesses. It is a feature of HIV infection that it clusters in families with often both parents HIV-positive (who in time experience morbidity and mortality). There is thus enormous strain on the capacity of families to cope with psycho-social and economic consequences of illness, such that many families experience great distress and often disintegrate as social and economic units.'

The localised evidence of such disintegration needs to be incorporated into national assessments of the cost to impoverished people of HIV/AIDS and the cost-benefits of delivering the services and material support that are so urgently needed.

**Child-headed households**
There is very limited information on child-headed households. Households may be headed by employed adult siblings of orphans, by school-going older siblings, by children caring for each other with adult support from another household, or by children caring for a dying parent with no adult support. The Children's Rights Centre in Durban stresses the need for more reliable information on the whereabouts and situation of orphaned children in order to assess vulnerability and need for support. In cases where a child has become a caregiver to an adult with HIV/AIDS, childhood is effectively sacrificed. As the adult mortality rate peaks there are likely to be many more households of this nature. Already some community organisations find themselves offering

training and support to children who are fulfilling adult roles at the expense of their own security and development. A strategy for government and community support that does not require children to become terminal care providers under the euphemism of home-based care is urgently needed.

**Children on the streets**
It is estimated that 10 000 children live or work on the streets in South Africa (ACESS, 2001). The Street Children's Forum in Durban runs shelters for children. Its Director, Julia Zingu, says they do not have data on children affected by AIDS but have seen a sharp increase in the numbers of children coming to the shelters. In addition, she notes that whereas before they were dealing with a single child from a family, they are increasingly accommodating whole families of siblings. Many of the children are working in the sex industry. Zingu said that the number of children living on the street had increased by almost 45 per cent between 1999 and 2000 and provided the following statistics on numbers of children living in first phase shelters:

　　1997:　1 405
　　1998:　1 268
　　1999:　1 587
　　2000:　2 554

This increase, and the increase in child prostitution, may reflect deepening poverty in families affected by AIDS, rising adult mortality due to AIDS and rising stress upon the extended family.

The role of AIDS in driving children out of the household, onto the streets or into commercial sex work should be further investigated, alongside the support mechanisms that might prevent or further delay such a move.

**Child abuse and neglect**
Child abuse, including sexual and physical abuse, increased by 117 per cent between 1993 and 1996. In 1998 there were approximately 34 000 reports of crimes against children including rape, incest, kidnapping, etc. (ACESS, 2001).

The prevalence and incidence of HIV and the risk factors for transmission mean that sexually abused children face a high risk of infection. While child abuse occurs across all socio-economic and cultural groups, when sexual abuse is reported, children from poor homes are most unlikely to be offered Voluntary Counselling and Testing (VCT). Government provision of post-exposure prophylaxis for rape survivors has to date been refused by Government. Apart from the trauma of abuse, the poorest children thus face the highest risk of HIV infection and the least possibility of access to preventive or life-saving medication. Abuse and neglect of children in AIDS-affected households is an indicator of the reduced ability of adults to cope. This increased vulnerability, and possible responses to it, is also an area where research seems to be minimal

## *Measures to reduce the impacts of HIV/AIDS on child poverty*
**Family/community responses**
The main measures to reduce the impacts of HIV/AIDS on children has clearly been taken by AIDS-affected households, who have drawn most of the country's orphans so far created into their extended families and cared at home for those dying from AIDS-related illnesses. While community workers in different parts of the country see some remaining capacity for absorbing orphans, the support structures on which extended family or community fostering depends are already under severe strain. Family responses tend to focus on survival but are holistic in as much as they do not isolate HIV/AIDS from other shocks and risks – they have to deal with threats relating to AIDS, unemployment, crime, etc. all at the same time.

**Civil society responses**
Among the main responses by AIDS support organisations to the problems faced by AIDS-affected and infected children are to:

- mobilise caregivers in the community to support the affected children;
- provide training and support to caregivers;
- assist caregivers and children to access welfare grants;
- assist caregivers and children to access services;
- lobby and fundraise around the additional needs of children affected by AIDS and poverty.

The first task is central to the survival and wellbeing of the child but its achievements are increasingly dependent on organisations delivering in all the other areas.

Many community-based projects have started out with a specific HIV/AIDS focus but have developed a holistic approach given the spectrum of crisis facing AIDS-affected children. Confronted by huge gaps in service delivery, they are often over-stretched in terms of the range of AIDS-affected children's needs – from food security to medication, education to foster care. One response to this overloading has been networking initiatives, like CINDI and ACESS.

**Government responses**
The responses of government to the HIV/AIDS epidemic have been multi-faceted. In this section emphasis will be on the formal institutional actions which government have in place to assist children generally and those actions

undertaken specifically in response to the epidemic. In particular, the impact of the epidemic on the existing welfare system to respond in a manner which is conducive to the optimal care of all children is closely examined.

**Existing welfare measures for children**
Well over half of children live in poverty and research suggests that this number is increasing, at least partly as a result of the HIV/AIDS epidemic (Institute for Democracy in South Africa, 2000). The burden of poverty is one of the biggest problems that children infected/affected by HIV/AIDS face. The government's poverty alleviation measures include the allocation of social assistance in the form of cash grants, to the caregivers of children who qualify in terms of certain criteria. At present, social assistance is solely the responsibility of the Department of Welfare.

While there are no special provisions for children infected/affected by HIV/AIDS, these children can access some financial support in the form of the child support grant (CSG) or foster grant (FG). The lengthy processing of grant applications usually means that the child/caregiver lacks support during a time when material and psycho-social support is critical. For adults in the terminal stages of AIDS, a disability grant is available. For children with full-blown AIDS, there are no special provisions available although some caregivers have managed to access the care dependency grant.

**Child support grant (CSG)**
The child support grant is targeted at poor children aged six years and under. The amount of R110 per month per child is provided, subject to a means test based on the personal income of the caregiver. The caregiver and child qualify if they live in:

An urban area:
- in a formal dwelling and the personal income is below R9 600 per annum;
- in an informal dwelling and the personal income is below R13 200 per annum.

A rural area:
- in a formal or informal dwelling and the personal income is below R13 200 per annum.

To access the CSG, the caregiver must present the bar-coded birth certificate of the child and their bar-coded identification document to the provincial Department of Social Development. Because HIV/AIDS is throwing increasing numbers of children below the income poverty line, the epidemic is making growing numbers of children eligible for the grant.

The grant is being phased in over a period of five years, between 1998 and 2003, with the target coverage being three million children. The target was based on estimates of the number of children living in poverty and does not take into account the impact of HIV/AIDS. Other estimates of the number of children under six years of age who qualify for the grant in terms of the means test are as high as double the department's figure of three million (Haarmann, 2001). The target of three million set by the department is used to determine the budget allocated to the grant. In spite of this, national and provincial statistics reveal that the budgetary allocations for the CSG do not match the projected targets. In KwaZulu-Natal for example, the provincial budget for the CSG was exceeded even though they only had a take up rate of 53 per cent of the targeted number of children (Child Health Policy Institute and Black Sash, 2000). If the budget for child and family grants is not substantially increased many children and families will not receive assistance.

> Two of Thembikile Shezi's daughters died of AIDS, each leaving five children for her to raise. Her eldest daughter is also dying and has left another eight children. Several of these children have tested HIV-positive. The family's plight is made worse by the fact that most of these children do not have birth certificates and Thembikile does not even know the names of the children's fathers. She does not have money to go to the nearest town, Pietermaritzburg, to have the children registered. Without birth certificates, she cannot apply for financial assistance. Even with the correct documents, she will only be able to apply for grants for a maximum of 6 of the 16 children. 'When the older children come home from school they cook, take care of the younger ones, and do the washing and ironing. When we had no food they never complained and on many nights I had to make them sleep with an empty stomach ... even the babies used to sleep without crying'
> 
> *Natal Witness*, 5 July 2000

The means test for accessing the CSG discriminates against larger households and will therefore discourage families from taking in AIDS orphans. The income of the primary caregiver has to be below a certain amount, regardless of how many children are dependent on that caregiver. Furthermore, it is only payable in respect of a maximum of 6 children per household. The grant therefore does not offer much assistance to families/grandparents caring for large numbers of young children.

Despite the fact that any adult primary caregiver, including the child's biological parents, may apply for the grant, the current uptake of the CSG is, at best, 33 per cent of the targeted three million. This is due in part to the difficulty in accessing the grant. Applicants must know the child's identification number and the parent's identification number, and must have proof of guardianship and a copy of the child's clinic card. Administrative delays in processing grant applications, poor attitude of administrative personnel, lack of knowledge of the available grants among communities, inaccessibility of grant application offices in rural areas, together with the fact that 51 per cent of children do not have birth certificates, means that many families living in desperate poverty are still denied the grant (Child Health Policy Institute and Black Sash, 2000).

**Foster grant (FG)**

For children who have been formally placed in the care of foster parents, through a children's court, a foster grant of R410 per month is available. There is also a means test for eligibility. The annual income of the foster child must not exceed twice the annual foster child grant. Only children that have been placed in the care of foster parents by a court of law are eligible for the grant. Each foster parent or parents can access grants for a maximum of six children. Increasing numbers of children will become eligible for this grant as courts place increasing numbers of children affected by HIV/AIDS in foster care. The amount of the foster grant is almost four times greater than the child support grant, thereby providing a disproportionate amount of support to caregivers who are not the biological parents of the child, and to the small minority of alternative caregivers who have gone through the lengthy process of formal fostering. There are at present approximately 72 000 children in foster care (President's Report, 1999). With an estimated 300 000 AIDS orphans in 2002, and an expected three million more within the next ten years, it can be expected that the demand on the foster care system will increase dramatically.

Foster care is an expensive model of care and placements have to be reviewed every two years. Apart from the actual monetary cost of the grant to the government, there is also the cost associated with children's court inquiries, statutory supervision services and grant administration.

While service providers warn of the impending crisis in the child and youth care system, the current formula for provincial budgetary planning does not include reference to the foster child grant. Provincial welfare budget allocations are calculated on the basis of the old age pension, disability grant and child support grant (i.e. children aged six years and under). The government therefore appears to be basing its budgetary planning on the assumption that caregivers of AIDS orphans will not be applying for the FG.

## Care dependency grant (CDG)
Children with severe disabilities are eligible for a care dependency grant of R570 per child, per month. The means test for this grant is that the combined annual income of the family, after deductions must not exceed R48 000 per annum.

This grant is for children with severe mental or physical disabilities, who require permanent home care. There is no specific provision for children with chronic illnesses, including HIV/AIDS. Few children in the terminal stages of AIDS have managed to access this grant but no formal policy exists to guide practitioners on whether and when HIV-positive children may be awarded this grant.

The majority of infections in children under the age of 13 years are through vertical transmission from mother to child. The child's HIV-positive status therefore implies that at least one of his/her parents is also HIV-positive. The impact on the family of a child's HIV-positive diagnosis can therefore be devastating with immediate and long-term socio-economic consequences.

In children, the interval between infection and mortality is compressed when compared to the same interval in adults, and the child's prognosis is dependent on a number of factors, including socio-economic conditions and nutritional status (Child Health Unit, 1998). These factors make it imperative that young children who are diagnosed as HIV-positive are given as much support as possible, as soon as possible. The CDG could offer these children the support they need.

## Treatment for HIV-positive children
While the Government's HIV/AIDS Directorate has issued guidelines for treatment of patients with AIDS-related illness, based on an Essential Drug List, AIDS support organisations in KwaZulu-Natal and the national advocacy organisation the Treatment Action Campaign (TAC) say that few, if any, of these treatments are available through the public health system. For example, in June 2001 the supplies of diflucin (fluconazole) donated by Pfizer for free treatment of HIV/AIDS-related life-threatening fungal infections, had not been distributed to hospitals and clinics. This means that poor households caring for someone with HIV/AIDS are paying for medication that is in theory available free, or are caring for a sick or dying person without any medication to treat symptoms or relieve pain.

Legislation passed by Parliament in 1997 (Amendment to the Medicines and Related Substances Act), allowing parallel importation and generic substitution to improve access to healthcare services was held up by the Pharmaceutical Manufacturers Association (PMA) court case until April 2001, when the PMA withdrew. However, the Health Minister has since announced that she is pursuing the longer-term option of local manufacture over importation, which could have begun immediately. For a child to be living with AIDS with no access to medication during sickness, pain and death is a complete denial of the right to survival, protection and development.

The most obvious way to protect children from the impoverishing impacts of HIV/AIDS is to prevent them from becoming orphaned or infected. This means providing affordable access to comprehensive medical treatment, including anti-retroviral (ARV) therapy for the prevention of mother to child transmission (MTCT) and to improve and prolong the lives of those infected. While government resistance to ARV has been developed from all angles, the objection in terms of affordability needs to be addressed. Given the measurable and immeasurable costs of AIDS to the next generation and the country, the cost-effectiveness and long-term cost-benefits of treatment need to be calculated.

**Care of orphans**

Government policy with regard to the care of AIDS orphans, according to Deputy Director of HIV/AIDS in the Department of Social Services and Population, Sakina Mohammed, is to concentrate on 'empowering the community to take care of orphans'. The government has placed a moratorium on setting up new children's homes and is concentrating instead on foster care.

The Government has committed line ministries to providing a continuum of care for vulnerable children and expresses commitment to integrating HIV/AIDS care and support across sectors. However, there is little co-ordination at national or provincial level and at grassroots level, there is fragmentation at best and non-delivery at worst.

Linda Aadnesgaard says of Thandanani's target communities: 'When children are left, it is often with a grandmother who very often can't get a birth certificate and then can't get access to benefits. Where there are clinics, there are still issues of access and proximity; children don't get treated without a blue card. Government officials' treatment of poor people is appalling. Our experience is that apart from the odd stalwart, children are treated with a lack of compassion and certainly not as a priority. So a poor grandmother with several children to care for has to try to access a system that is very unfriendly. The distance and time that grannies, and everyone, have to go to seek medical care is absolutely killing. The nurses are rude, there is no medication and if you have three different conditions you have to go on three different days.'

While studies have been done in other countries (Zambia, Tanzania, Zimbabwe, etc.) on the comparative costs of home-based care (HBC) and hospital-based care of HIV/AIDS patients, these have tended to look at cost to the government. There is local empirical evidence of the coping strategies and the limits to the coping strategies used by impoverished families strained further by HIV/AIDS (e.g. CINDI, Thandanani, in KwaZulu-Natal; Siyawela, Soweto; Homes of Hope, Mpumalanga). There do not seem to be any extensive studies or analyses that could inform inter-sectoral responses – including budgets – nationally. Research is needed into:

- potential comparative cost of HBC to the government;
- actual costs of HBC – material, time, emotional, opportunity – to a household (children and adults);
- factors that determine whether the household absorbs or breaks under the burden;
- cost-benefit to the household and the government of an integrated approach to supporting the household in meeting those costs, through effective delivery of existing and enhanced social grants to children living in poverty;
- short- and long-term costs to children and the country of failing to provide such support.

Children's rights and welfare organisations nationally argue that ensuring access to existing benefits (pensions, disability grants and child support or foster care grants) is an essential and urgent step, while implementing a Basic Income Grant and targeting special assistance to especially vulnerable children would help to offset some of the impoverishing effects of HIV/AIDS.

Smart (1999) draws out lessons and limitations of model projects with regard to exactly these issues. Most of the lessons relate to the importance of an holistic and integrated approach to prevention and care of all affected family members, to the importance of training to equip family and community members to provide care, and to the importance of social security against a background of deep poverty. Most of the limitations relate to the scale of need, which families and community organisations simply can't meet, and to limited access to medication, services and social grants, regardless of availability and eligibility.

Ninety-four per cent of institutional places for children have been closed but there has not been a proportionate shift in funding to support foster care. A subsidy of R510 is available to families fostering a child but this is difficult for many caregivers to access. Johannesburg's Child Welfare co-ordinator, Jackie Loffel, agrees with the emphasis on fostering but says the policy has not been thought through carefully: 'It is a myth to think that because less money is spent on children's homes that there is more available for spending on foster care'.

Where a family is affected by AIDS, the absence of welfare is acutely impoverishing. Young children orphaned and left in the care of a grandmother or other extended family member face more obstacles to securing a CSG than other children. There have been cases where a CSG 'was denied because the surname of the child on the Road to Health card was not the same as the caregiver's' (ACESS, 2001). This situation, and problems with securing birth certificates and accessing foster care grants, is increasingly common due to parental deaths from AIDS.

## Conclusion

HIV/AIDS is acknowledged to have an impoverishing effect on every aspect of children's lives. The need for a holistic, integrated approach to address this is stressed by most. However, the impacts felt by children at household and community level, even where documented by local organisations, are rarely integrated into research, policy and programme planning around HIV/AIDS and poverty.

A rights-based approach to treatment issues – both for infected children and for their caregivers – needs to be developed to ensure an holistic approach to alleviating child poverty. Access to treatment, from nutrition supplements, to alternative care, to anti-retroviral therapy is a neglected issue in terms of child survival and the rights to equality, dignity and family care.

The knowledge of AIDS support and service organisations, of the capacity, costs and support needs related to home-based and community-based care should provide the basis for urgent allocation of resources to strengthen that care.

Current debates about affordability and cost-effectiveness of different models of care are highly politicised. Urgent delivery of appropriate services would be facilitated by reliable data on the savings through reducing HIV/AIDS care in health facilities and the full range of costs to children and their communities.

The impact of HIV/AIDS on child poverty should not be assessed on the basis of statistics or analysed only by adults. Further research to support effective interventions on behalf of children needs to listen to children's voices.

## References

Alliance for Children's Entitlement to Social Security. 2001. *Children, HIV and Poverty*. Cape Town.

Caelers, D. and L. Johns. 2001. 'Education Faces AIDS Nightmare'. *Cape Argus*. 28 February.

Child Health Policy Institute. 2001. 'Workshop Report: National Workshop on Social Security for Children in South Africa'. March. University of Cape Town, Cape Town.

Child Health Policy Institute and Black Sash. 2000. 'Issue Paper on Social Security for Children in South Africa'. Report prepared for the Commission of Enquiry into a Comprehensive Social Security System in South Africa. University of Cape Town, Cape Town.

Child Health Unit. 1998. *HIV/AIDS and the Family: A Clinical Guide*. Cape Town: University of Cape Town.

Cohen, D. 2000. 'Poverty and HIV/AIDS in Sub-Saharan Africa'. Paper presented to conference of Social Development and Poverty Elimination Division of the United Nations Development Program, June.

*Daily Dispatch*. 2001. 'Children Starve as Social Grants System Fails'. 19 April.

*Daily Dispatch*. 2001. 'Over 80% in EC Hungry: Survey'. 25 April.

Department of Welfare 2001. *National Workshop on Social Security for Children in South Africa*. Pretoria.

Department of Welfare and Population Development 1997. *White Paper for Social Welfare*. Pretoria.

Haarmann, C. 2001. *Social Assistance in South Africa: Its Potential Impact on Poverty*. PhD thesis, University of the Western Cape, Cape Town.

Institute for Democracy in South Africa. 2000. *Child Poverty and the Budget*. Cape Town: Budget Information Service.

Institute for Democracy in South Africa. 2002. 'The Child Support Grant and Budget 2002'. *Budget Brief 2002*. Cape Town: Budget Information Service.

Loffell, J. and C. Phiroshaw. 2001. 'Child Labour: Sitting on the Statistics Won't Solve the Problem'. *Children FIRST* 5(36): 8.

Marcus, T. 1999. *Wo! Zaphela Izingane – It is Destroying the Children: Living and Dying with AIDS*. Pietermaritzburg: Children in Distress (CINDI) Network.

The Presidency. 1999. *President's Report on the State of the Nation's Children*. Pretoria.

Smart, R. 1999. *Children Living with HIV/AIDS in South Africa: A Rapid Appraisal*. Johannesburg: Save the Children.

UNAIDS. 2000. *Report on the Global HIV/AIDS Epidemic: June 2000*. Geneva: United Nations.

Whiteside, A. (ed.). 1998. *Implications of AIDS for Demograph and Policy in Southern Africa*. Pietermaritzburg: University of Natal Press.

CHAPTER 5

# Education

*Peter Badcock-Walters*

## Background
This chapter seeks to analyse the impact of HIV/AIDS on the education of children in South Africa, and examines two broad areas of concern. First, it considers the problems of access to education, and analyses the factors influencing this; specifically, focusing on the impact of infections and death of parents. Second, it examines the impact of HIV/AIDS on educators and other officials in management and administration, and attempts to demonstrate the affect of this on delivery and maintenance of education services.

## The education context
The process of education and learning is the key to social, cultural and political participation, personal and community economic empowerment, and national development. Its output is the human capital which constitutes the nation's primary wealth and potential for growth.

Anything that threatens or diminishes the role of education directly impacts and reduces personal, community and national development and, in fact, reverses previous gains. HIV/AIDS represent the largest single threat to this education process, by increasing the scale of almost every existing problem of supply, quality and output. Moreover, this threat is increased exponentially by a general lack of recognition of the seriousness of the problem and its impact on the systemic functioning of education at all levels. To place this in perspective, it should be noted that one-third of all HIV-infected persons were infected during their school years, while a further third were infected within two years of leaving school. This confirms schools as a high-risk environment but also suggests that it is the key strategic ground on which the battle to mitigate the impact will be won or lost.

HIV/AIDS is the wild card that entirely confounds the rational business of education planning and management. In general terms the education system has yet to come to terms with the fact that HIV/AIDS is a development issue and, by definition, the key management challenge facing the system. Instead it continues to be erroneously regarded as a health issue, albeit serious, that has crossed the path of education development, and one that largely requires curriculum change, improved sexual and reproductive health education, materials development and condom distribution to resolve or at least mitigate its impact.

Clearly, an adequate response to the threat of HIV/AIDS requires both a systemic and sustainable management response and the parallel address and improvement of appropriate curricula, sexual and reproductive health education and relevant materials development, in order to effect behaviour change. Irrespective of the quality of curricula and education-driven interventions, the success of these will be limited by the structural stability and comparative functionality of the system.

It is obvious, in this regard, that teachers whose personal behaviour and standards of discipline are questionable, will not be appropriate role models or indeed credible communicators on subjects such as low risk behaviour and informed personal choice. Nor are such teachers likely to reform or improve their own behaviour if the school in which they teach is inadequately or ineffectively managed and disciplined.

For the public education system to survive as an effective delivery mechanism for teaching and learning, it is simply vital that its administrators take a long-term view of the impact of HIV/AIDS. The existing high attrition rates for educators and managers will be exacerbated directly as a result of morbidity and mortality in the system, and indirectly by recruitment from other affected sectors. Consequent conditions and service ratios may therefore condemn declining cohorts of learners to deteriorating quality and standards of achievement, for the foreseeable future. This situation can, however, be mitigated – to a greater or lesser extent – through recognition and understanding, enlightened planning, management reform and improved classroom practice and school discipline.

## *Access to education: The impact of illness and death in the home*

In attempting to analyse problems of access arising from HIV infections and the AIDS death(s) of parents in the home, it is necessary to make the point that the impact of HIV/AIDS exacerbates the scale of existing management problems. In the case of access, it is important to recognise that it has always been a major problem for the education system.

According to the 1996 Census there were an estimated 1.3 million children between the ages of seven and 18 out of school, with the provinces of the Eastern Cape and KwaZulu-Natal the worst affected (Statistics South Africa, 1996). There is however no information on the reasons for this figure, which is equal to more than ten per cent of the enrolled school population.

Thus the advent of HIV infection in the home, followed by AIDS-related mortality, will build on already high levels of voluntary or enforced exclusion, aggravating the impact on education and contributing to the decline in enrolments, transition rates and output from the system.

**The impact of HIV-related illness in the home**
The incidence of HIV infection in the home can be expected to further reduce access to education, due to increased economic hardship, family care and other household or agrarian duties, the need to find employment, declining health due to deteriorating nutrition and other opportunistic infections, and the effects of personal trauma associated with grief, stress and added responsibility.

In the context of this analysis, the development of HIV or AIDS-related illness is likely to have profound consequences for the home life of the learner on both a physical and psychological level, including the possible impact of ostracisation and marginalisation.

In terms of access for the children of infected parents, there are a number of direct and indirect issues arising.

First, infected adults are likely to begin a cycle of absenteeism, both short- and medium-term, from their places of employment. For a self-employed person, this will preclude the individual from earning a livelihood for variable periods of time. This would constitute a direct blow to the economic viability of the household, and place increased demands on its limited reserves, for healthcare and income replacement. This constraint on employment and economic activity will inevitably reduce the capacity of the household to support children in school. With competing priorities for limited resources, children living in AIDS-affected households are often unable to afford school uniforms, school fees and textbooks and other materials or provide the financial resources required for transport and school feeding. Children who are unable to pay school fees report being expelled from school, being held back a grade, having report cards withheld, being threatened by teachers, being excluded from the school feeding scheme and being embarrassed and teased (Giese, Proudlock and Meintjes, 2002).

Poverty and education access are therefore inextricably linked; for example, research in 1993 indicated that more than two-thirds of individuals living in households whose head had completed less than four years of formal education, were living in poverty (Education Foundation, EduAction and Whiteford 2000).

Second, as the cycle of illness develops, the breadwinner or parent concerned may require nursing and direct physical and emotional support on a more or less constant basis. As a consequence, the school-going child may be cast in the role of caregiver and nurse, or income earner, and may – in extreme cases – be coerced into crime or prostitution in order to contribute to the very survival of the household. It is arguably such economic deprivation that contributes to the cycle of opportunistic sexual encounters so commonly observed (the Sugar Daddy syndrome) throughout sub-Saharan Africa, and which are often seen as a means of survival and of financing access to education.

But would these stresses necessarily preclude a child from access to schooling? In short, the inability to pay school fees may indeed prohibit the entry of the child to school. While there is clear and articulate national policy insisting that every child has the right of access, school principals are faced with issues of institutional viability and routinely turn away learners unable to pay fees. Even if the school was to permit entry, the fact is that the child would be hard pressed to pay for stationery and textbooks, as well as transport and food at school.

Third, arising from this identification with illness in the home, the issue of stigmatisation in the community and marginalisation in the school is a very real barrier to access and participation. While levels of awareness of HIV/AIDS are patently high, so too are levels of suspicion and fear. Thus a child coming from a home in which infection is perceived to be HIV linked, may be stigmatised or even physically deterred from entry to school by his or her peers, or simply so traumatised by the reaction that they themselves opt to stay away.

The question also arises of the potential for support from the extended family system and which remains a key source of hope in the absence of a formal social security system. What is clear is that this traditional system of support functions very effectively when one member of an extended family network experiences difficulty, financial or otherwise. But in the face of the unprecedented impact of HIV/AIDS, the equation may change, many members of the extended family network may now be infected or affected, and consequently, the capacity of the network to react is badly compromised by the multiple impacts upon it. The net effect of this comparative disablement of community support systems will be to limit the capacity of sources outside the affected home to assist.

These physical constraints on the child in an affected home would in themselves be enough to deter continuing participation and suggest that the child would be too busy to attempt to maintain the learning process. In addition to these very real barriers to access, the child will also be exposed to extreme levels of personal insecurity and trauma. This will occur in circumstances beyond the reach or support of those few councillors and welfare officers available to the system, and will expose the child to intolerable pressures that may preclude effective learning even if he or she continues to attend school.

In the event of the death of a parent, for any reason, the child is equally but more permanently affected. However, if one parent dies of an AIDS-related opportunistic disease, the chances are good that the surviving parent will also fall ill and later succumb. Thus in addition to the physical loss, the loss of income, the insecurity and the associated trauma, the child may well anticipate a repeat cycle in the household and even some degree of social stigma. If it is the child's mother who has died, or indeed if both parents have died, the child becomes an orphan by technical definition and faces an uncertain future. The child may well find him or herself the *de facto* household head, perhaps responsible for younger siblings, and without the means or time to continue in school. The net effect of these circumstances may be to drive the child from school and into a life of servitude or obligation (either within an extended family environment or outside it), into employment or unemployment, perhaps involving a life of crime or prostitution as a survival strategy.

The bleakness of this scenario does not require amplification. On one level the child's learning path will be substantially or permanently disrupted, and even if it is not, he or she will have to continue their school life in circumstances of extreme deprivation and personal trauma.

All of the issues identified above in respect of illness in the home continue to be problems in the context of the death of one or both parents, which may be seen as the termination of a debilitating cycle of attrition and dependence. The singular difference is that there may be a sense of closure, and even some measure of physical and emotional release insofar as home care and other obligations may be ended. However, these may be replaced by other, more complex social dynamics that may, for example, have the affect of physically uplifting the child into a new environment (an extended family or other foster home), casting them in the role of an un/under-resourced household head or alternatively displacement from any home or shelter. The key dynamic is this regard is the classification of the child as an orphan, and their increased vulnerability in society.

Projections suggest about one in five children of school-going age will be orphaned by 2010. The issue of access will become increasingly important to a level that is unprecedented, and may mean that orphaned children constitute an entire generation of educational disenfranchised young people. It is likely that they will drop in and out of the system at an increased rate and may not be retained long enough to graduate either the primary or secondary phase, thus impacting output, tertiary access and educated entry into the world of work.

In summary, the child in an affected household, with an infected parent to consider and even care for, will be exposed to a variety of impacts that together may reduce or even preclude access to schooling, either temporarily or permanently. It is therefore important to see this problem in the context of a number of related and contributory factors.

## Correlation between HIV infection and school enrolment rates
HIV prevalence rates in national terms are extremely high by any criteria.

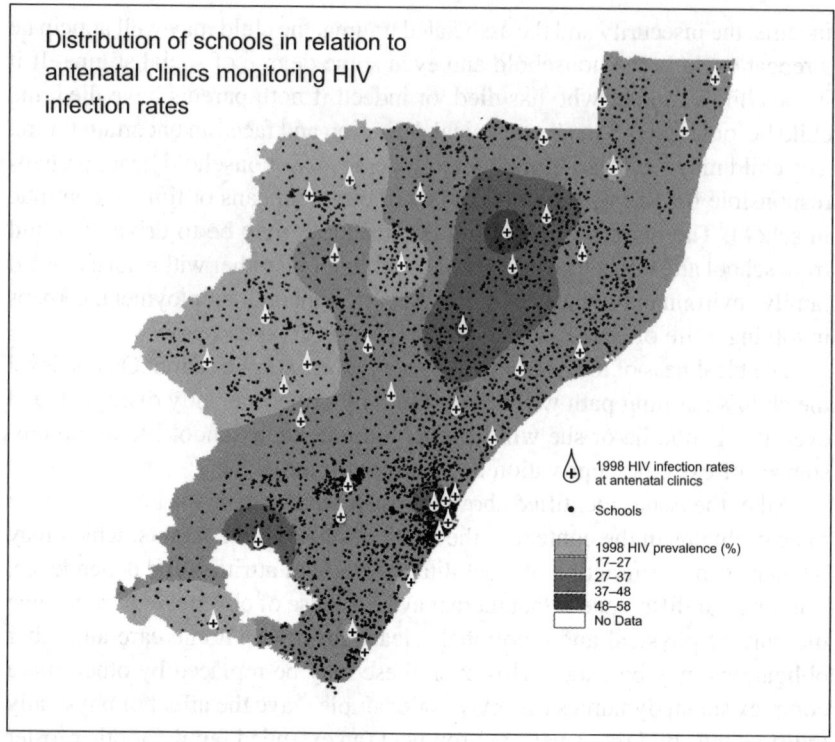

Figure 5.1  **Relationship between HIV infection and enrolment rates.**

However, the rates for the country's nine provinces show variable levels of infection. Overall however, the data confirms the dramatic impact of the disease in every province.

In these circumstances, it is reasonable to conclude that the scale of impact on households, and therefore on children in school (and out of it), is likely to be enormous. In simplistic terms it is reasonable to suppose that at least one in every four homes will be directly affected, increasing to one in every three in the worst affected provinces, such as KwaZulu-Natal, Mpumalanga, Gauteng and the Free State which between them constitute over half of the total South African population. Prevalence continues to peak amongst the most economically active segment of this population (aged 20–39) confirming the extent of the problem facing households and the school-going children in them.

One important point should be noted however. These national and provincial statistics mask the fact that there is very considerable geographic variation in prevalence rates, and therefore in levels of impact on schools districts and the learners in them. For example, in KwaZulu-Natal, antenatal prevalence rates vary from almost 60 per cent in clinics and hospitals in the north to less than a third of that figure in other areas (HEARD and EduAction, 2000). The point is, that with some exceptions, these antenatal prevalence hot spots coincide with areas of greatest economic deprivation, the under-provision of classrooms, schools and associated utilities as well as the incidence of poor nutrition and other endemic diseases (Figure 5.1).

**Declining enrolment**
While insufficient analysis of enrolment data has been done, there is already evidence in the province of KwaZulu-Natal of quite dramatic impact on enrolment in Grade 1. An analysis of Grade 1 enrolment indicates an historical growth of between three per cent and five per cent per annum over the last 20 years; however in 1999, a three per cent growth rate in 1998 reversed to a 12 per cent decline. In 2000, there was a further drop of 24 per cent, a decline exacerbated by regulations that precluded the entry of children under the age of seven from that year. In 2001, data indicates an increase in Grade 1 enrolment of 18 per cent, but this is in fact still 12 per cent short of the increase required to take up the anticipated holdover from the preceding year's regulatory change, and equates to a real decline of 12 per cent over the three year period (Badcock-Walters et al., 2001).

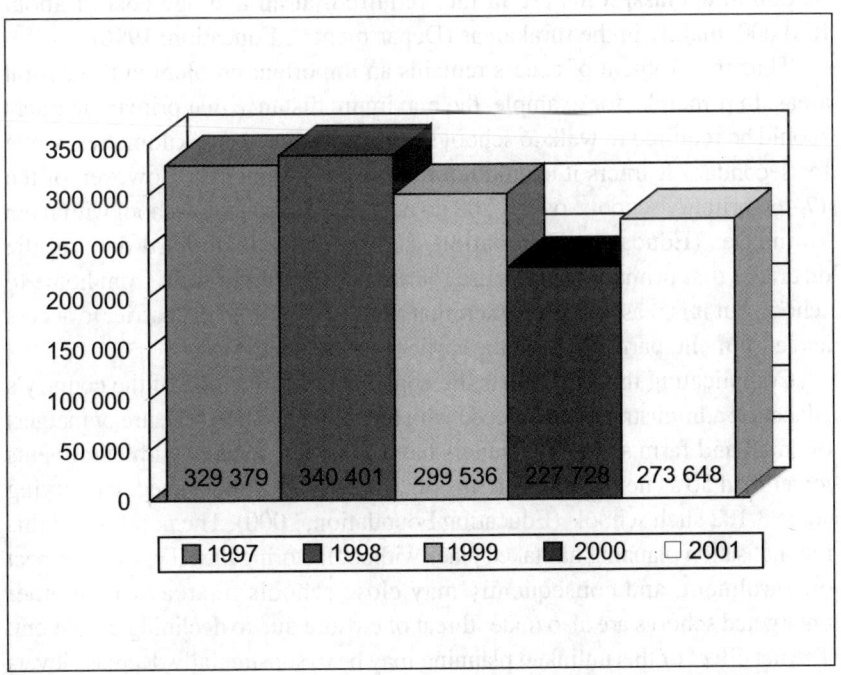

Figure 5.2   Grade 1 enrolment in KwaZulu-Natal (1997–2001).

In other words, in the South African province exhibiting the highest impact of HIV/AIDS prevalence, there is a dramatic and perhaps not coincidental decline in Grade 1 enrolment, which now means that there are fewer than 60 per cent of the number of learners in Grade 1 that there were in 1998. While there are many apparent reasons for this decline, most of these could be said to be directly or indirectly affected or exacerbated by HIV/AIDS, and confirm the extent of difficulties facing the education system.

**Physical infrastructure**

While there has been much work to reduce the inherited apartheid backlog, this has still fallen far short of the requirement for new and refurbished classrooms, particularly in relation to the rural areas of the former homelands of the country.

Learner enrolment is highest in the major metropolitan areas such as Johannesburg, Durban, and Port Elizabeth, and in the Magisterial Districts immediately adjacent to them. However, the distribution of the 27 500 schools (in 2000) does not coincide with the extent of rural demand and is often confounded by issues of geography and dynamic and unpredictable changes in human settlement patterns (Education Foundation, 2000). An estimated 58 000 new classrooms are in fact required, at an average cost of about R70 000, mainly in the rural areas (Department of Education, 1996).

Thus the problem of access remains an important problem in these rural areas. In principle, for example, the maximum distance that primary learners should be required to walk to school should not exceed five kilometres, while for secondary learners it should not exceed ten kilometres. However, of the 17 466 primary schools, over 3 200 do not have a secondary school within ten kilometres (Education Foundation, 2000). There is no hard data on the distances that primary learners are routinely expected to walk from home to school, but it is reasonable to assert that this constitutes a real barrier to access and enrolment, particularly in the earlier grades.

Complicating this problem is the apparent determination of the country's education administrators to proceed with the rationalisation (closure or merger) of small and farm schools. Planners have specified schools with enrolments lower than 50 as non-viable in terms of cost and educational need, identifying some 3 102 such schools (Education Foundation, 2000). The point is that this rationalisation planning has taken place without factoring the HIV/AIDS impact on enrolment, and consequently may close schools in areas where other untargeted schools are also under threat of closure due to declining enrolment. The net effect of this unlinked planning may be to substantially decrease levels of access over and above that anticipated in the rationalisation planning process, and to create education deserts in rural areas.

**Gender inequity and access**
South Africa has had, and to some extent continues to have, a unique level of gender equity in its schooling system, relative to its sub-Saharan neighbours. One obvious implication of the impact of HIV/AIDS on the home and school environment is that girls will be more affected than boys, and that this balance will be upset.

There are a number of reasons for this, and include the fact that girls are more likely to be withdrawn from school than boys, in the event of economic hardship and deprivation, and more likely to be held back to provide care both for the infected party and for siblings now without care themselves. Girls are also more likely than boys to become the victims of sexual exploitation in these circumstances and may in fact be driven to this course as a means of personal survival and household support. What can be said is that the research into declining Grade 1 enrolment in KwaZulu-Natal, cited above, has also shown a disproportionate decline in the enrolment of girls into the first year of school. There is also likely to be a decline in the number of girls matriculating and a consequent drop in the gross number of Matriculants.

## *The impact of HIV/AIDS on education delivery and maintenance*
Education delivery and maintenance will be significantly impacted by the illness and premature death of educators and officials at every level, and by the consequent erosion of systems and structures as a result of the loss of capacity, specialist skills and experience. Two distinct areas of impact will be evidenced, the first in the provision and replacement of educators in the classroom, and the second in the area of system management and administration, at all levels.

The first will have a profound effect on the business of teaching and learning, and may worsen learner/educator ratios, in spite of declining enrolment, and compromise both quality and output through loss of teaching experience. This impact will also prejudice prospects for positive behaviour change anticipated as a result of curriculum reform, materials development and appropriate role modelling.

The second area may be far more serious insofar as the potential for systemic failure is concerned, and may compromise administration and every aspect of education management, not least because the number of experienced managers and administrators available to the system is already extremely limited. While managers and administrators are theoretically less vulnerable to HIV/AIDS than their colleagues in the classroom, because of their higher average age, they are also closer to retirement and consequently replacement by younger officials, drawn from a higher-risk age-group and environment.

The health and performance of the system itself is therefore under threat, and while schools have a long-demonstrated ability to function without departmental support and guidance, the potential collapse of teaching and learning within the school represents a medium- to long-term crisis of unprecedented proportions.

### Key management issues

Several key management issues present themselves and should be viewed in the context of illness and death in the home, since the delivery and maintenance of education takes place in a community environment and is subject to its reflected stresses and concerns.

### Data and information

Data remains a problem and means that strategic planning – particularly at the provincial level – is largely informed by estimates, projections, anecdotal information and comparative country insights. Until 2000, when the first capture of educator and learner mortality rates was undertaken in the Annual Survey for the preceding year (1999), there was no data for prevalence, infection rates or mortality in these groups (National and Provincial Departments of Education, 2000). As will be seen below, however, these initial data may be unreliable, and will require further sampling and analysis. This aside, the system has not routinely collected data on the temporary and permanent loss of learners, educators and managers that provides sufficient detail to pinpoint the impact of HIV/AIDS beyond contention. In the absence of the systemic collection of data by government, several supplementary research activities have been undertaken.

### Temporary educator losses

The primary impact of HIV will be to increase the incidence and length of temporary educator absence due to illness, occasional and compassionate leave (for funerals and associated family trauma). This, together with the psychological impact of the illness, will reduce contact time, performance and quality, and will lead to increased health and replacement-educator costs in the system.

This impact may in fact be harder to measure and understand than permanent educator loss from the system, since it involves subtle degrees of absence ranging from complete physical absence, to attendance for some part of the teaching day, to physical disassociation and detachment from the teaching task, in spite of being physically present. Since most provincial systems neglect to keep or capture educator attendance records, this impact may be consistently underestimated and may be more damaging than more measurable permanent absence, in real terms, since it creates the assumption that teaching and learning are taking place.

## Educator and management attrition

The permanent loss of educators and managers through death, relocation, employment change, retirement or chronic illness is already very high, confirming that HIV/AIDS will exacerbate existing attrition rates. In KwaZulu-Natal, the largest provincial system with over 71 000 publicly-paid educators, attrition rates were at 6.7 per cent in 1999, only one per cent of which was directly AIDS-attributable. This equated to the loss of 5 300 educators in that year, of whom only around 750 were estimated to have died as a direct result of AIDS (Crouch, 2001).

There is evidence that educators – and perhaps managers – are more HIV prevalent than the general population they serve, possibly for reasons of comparatively high income, social status and mobility, and positions of power over large numbers of learners.

Data on educator mortality was captured for the first time in 2000, for the 1999 education year. The results for KwaZulu-Natal, the first province to be analysed, reflect such an improbably dramatic impact that further research is required. Only 471 of 5 972 schools submitted returns on the question of educator deaths from illness during 1999, reporting 424 deaths from a sample of 6 553 educators employed in the schools concerned (KwaZulu-Natal Department of Education and Culture, 2001). These preliminary results indicate mortality rates of 8.4 per cent in the sample of 2 282 males, and 5.5 per cent in the sample of 4 271 females (aged 20 to 60); mortality peaked between 30–34 for females and 35–39 for males. These rates are so far ahead of any projection or trend that there is some doubt that the data could be accurate, and may be the result of misunderstanding of the apparently very clear question. However, what it does confirm is that there are a significant number of deaths from illness amongst educators under the age of 50, an incidence generally taken to be a proxy for AIDS mortality.

## Educator training

Existing attrition rates will be further impacted by AIDS mortality and demand for new educators will grow – indeed quite dramatically – in spite of shrinking enrolment. In a sector that employs over 350 000 educators, with attrition rates running as high as seven per cent in some areas, this will have considerable financial and institutional implications, particularly since national government has recently closed its Educator Training Colleges and transferred responsibility for this function to the University sector. Growing prevalence rates in student intakes will also be a significant factor.

In KwaZulu-Natal alone, it is estimated that over 60 000 new educators will be required by 2010, simply to hold educator/learner ratios at their present high levels. This equates to almost the total number of publicly-paid educators presently in that system, and would require the universities in that province to increase their gross student intake by over 50 per cent (Provincial Education Development Unit, 2001). This raises several important policy issues, including the possibility that educators may have to be trained in less than three years in order to meet this escalating demand.

**Delivery planning**
The planning of delivery and services will in future have to integrate the impact of both HIV and AIDS in every aspect of activity and budgeting, with mid-level impact scenarios the probable default position until more reliable data is available. The planning of the renovation and building of classrooms and schools will require fresh appraisal of local demographics, for example, as will the rationalisation and merger of under-utilised facilities, such as small and farm schools. The provision of potable water, sanitation and health and counselling services will take on a new significance and may reorder planners' traditional priorities and goals.

It can no longer be business as usual, given that in some districts enrolments may decline to less than half their historical levels in some grades, yet still exhibit unacceptably high learner/educator ratios due to teacher morbidity and mortality. The way in which educators are posted for example, often far from home districts and separate from a teaching spouse, requires that a revised code of planning practice be developed and adopted, to minimise the exposure of the system, first to traditional management and administrative failure and, second, to the increase in these problems stemming from HIV/AIDS impact.

**Service ratios**
While enrolment, and therefore demand, is set to decline for the foreseeable future, the supply of trained educators will decline even faster due to existing attrition, direct AIDS impact and the indirect affect of increased competitive demand in the wider workplace due to AIDS-related deaths in the workforce. Thus, learner/educator ratios will worsen in many areas over time, but as importantly, declining quality due to the loss of qualified and experienced educators will also occur. Even where these ratios may appear acceptable, educators may not be functioning effectively and may mask deeper problems of contact and quality. Ironically, learner/classroom ratios may also worsen due to small school rationalisation and the inevitable effect of multi-grading, necessitated by the temporary or permanent absence of educators. In these circumstances, community and other un/under-qualified volunteers may also make an appearance in the classroom, particularly in rural areas, to assist until such time as replacements are available.

The ratio of qualified to un/under-qualified educators may also not improve as expected, for the reasons outlined above, not least because educators – including scarce specialised subject educators – appear to be equally at risk irrespective of their qualifications.

**Declining fee income**
The Department of Education has been very successful in developing a method of 'Resource Targeting' to identify the poorest schools in the country and has established a means of redirecting resources to compensate for comparative and historical disadvantage. Notwithstanding this, pressure on household income will impact the payment of both compulsory and voluntary school fees and levies, and will reduce ability to pay for textbooks, uniforms, school lunches and transport. The net effect will be to render many schools insolvent, given that large numbers of these depend on this income for a range of expenses, from administration to extra educator salaries – often in order to maintain acceptable learner/educator ratios. There are already widespread reports from schools and School Governing Bodies in this regard, citing bankruptcy due to large-scale defaulting on payments by parents. Notwithstanding the government's commitment to provision and resourcing, it should be noted that these school and related fees can be extremely high, and it may become necessary to allocate emergency or supplementary funding to address the problem.

**Transition rates and output**
Drop out rates can be expected to increase, while quality in the classroom declines due to temporary and permanent educator absence and loss of contact time. This may mean that the number of learners making the transition from the primary to secondary phase may be expected to decline, or at the least, for the quality of those making the transition to decline. This impact will also be aggravated by the proportionally greater decline in the number of girls retained in the system, given that they have constituted the majority of learners in the higher grades.

This implies that the incremental improvement in Matriculation rates may be at risk and even reversed, both in terms of quality and quantity. Moreover, this may be a medium to long-term phenomena, since it is apparent that enrolment in the first grade is also showing real decline and that the system is contracting at an unexpectedly high rate. Output from the system, in the form of demand for tertiary and further education, has historically exceeded supply, but this demand may now be reduced both by the drop in the real number of learners qualifying for entrance and those able to pay for such higher education.

## Budget implications

To put these issues in context, it must be understood that education consumes almost a quarter of the national budget and employs or enrols almost a third of the country's population. Moreover, educator salaries account for well over 90 per cent of the education budget (Department of Education, 2001). This confirms that HIV/AIDS impact in this high-risk sector is of the greatest strategic and budgetary significance.

The fiscal impact of educator training on the scale evidenced in KwaZulu-Natal has yet to be understood or factored, but this is merely a line item relative to the problem of reduced system quality, output and volume of qualified entrants to the world of work. The real impact will be on consequent economic growth and national development, and will be felt for two to three decades to come. The key budget implication is that HIV/AIDS must be factored in every aspect of recurrent and capital expenditure, and must anticipate reduced income revenue and a slowing in anticipated rates of economic growth. What is therefore required is that management of the education budget is reviewed and redesigned to account for these impacts, at every level of the fiscal process.

## Strategic planning for management and mitigation: Next steps

Since 1994, there has developed a tradition of strategic planning that has led to the development of any number of visionary policies. The quality and depth of the Schools Act, the product of exhaustive consultation and strategic planning is a case in point, as is the more recently published policy on HIV/AIDS in education.

However, a widely acknowledged problem exists in the separation of powers between the national and provincial departments, with the latter being responsible for implementation. This often results in a disconnection between the expressed intent of the national Department of Education and the capacity and will of the provincial departments to implement and operationalise policies.

In the case of HIV/AIDS, a number of provincial departments have begun to react appropriately to the scale of the challenge, notably Gauteng and KwaZulu-Natal, with the latter commissioning a number of strategically important research initiatives, including an educator demand model, an analysis of declining enrolment and preliminary estimates of educator and learner mortality.

But few of these departments have the knowledge and capacity to take the design of countermeasures forward, and as a matter of the greatest urgency must initiate a review of their comparative circumstances and undertake a strategic planning process designed to manage and mitigate impact on their systems. While this should be done with the support and guidance of the national Department of Education, the fact remains that there are very considerable social, economic and educational differences between these provinces, as well as very variable levels of impact within them, and consequently suggests the need for targeted and specific intervention planning, within a principled national framework.

The important point is that they – individually and as a nationally coordinated and interdependent group of provinces – must recognise HIV/AIDS as the greatest management challenge facing their systems, and take appropriate steps to mitigate its impact. These include the review of policy and regulations, the initiation of a strategic planning process involving all key stakeholder groups, the creation of an enforceable regulatory framework, the capture and analysis of data to inform the position and the empowerment of managers at all levels to manage their way through what are traditional systemic problems, exploded in scale by HIV/AIDS. This will necessitate identifying all the stakeholders – allies and inhibitors – and engaging in multi-sectoral partnerships to deal comprehensively with the unprecedented scale of the crisis.

## *Conclusion*

Infected educators and managers may continue in the system – at declining levels of productivity – for another ten or fifteen years, dependent on levels of healthcare and support. Ultimately their loss will require the accelerated training of replacements, which will bring with it increased risk due to the lower average ages of these replacement educators and their comparative inexperience.

Learners will likewise graduate or drop out of this high-risk environment with a significant number already infected, and with an equivalent number likely to be infected within one or two years of leaving this system. Curriculum change, materials development and condom distribution, while apparently contributing to high levels of awareness, have shown little evidence of influencing behaviour to date. Prevailing social dynamics, peer pressure, economic circumstances and lack of positive role models, suggests that at least another generation may pass through the system before this pattern changes to any marked degree.

It is clear that the magnitude of this problem is beyond the experience of everyone involved. It is also clear that there are major psychological barriers obscuring its resolution and creating levels of personal stress and trauma that leave officials at every level apparently impotent in the face of the epidemic.

The challenge is to see beyond the system turbulence that lies ahead and plan for the kind of change that can only be countenanced in crisis; in short, to recognise in this state of emergency the opportunity to review and redesign the way, teaching and learning, and redirect the education system. There is widespread recognition of the shortcomings of the system and even greater recognition of an inability to do much about it – in normal circumstances. This opportunity in crisis should be grasped precisely because the national trauma that will develop around the impact of HIV/AIDS must be counterbalanced with the good news of improvement and reform. South Africa has the capacity to rise to this challenge, manage its way through this period of crisis and redesign its education future. What is required is recognition, vision, planning and political will.

**References**
Badcock-Walters, P., Provincial Education Development Unit (PEDU). 2001. *Where Have All the Flowers Gone?* Durban.
Crouch, L. 2001. *The District Education Management Information System: An Educator Demand/Supply Model.* Chapel Hill: Research Triangle Institute.
Department of Education. 1996. *School Register of Needs.* Pretoria.
Department of Education. 2001. *Education Budget Papers.* Pretoria.
Education Foundation, EduAction, Whiteford A. 2000. *The Education Atlas of South Africa 2000.* Education Foundation , Durban.
Giese, S., P. Proudlock and H. Meintjes. 2002. *Report on the National Children's Forum on HIV/AIDS.* Cape Town: Children's Institute, University of Cape Town.
Health Economics and HIV/AIDS Research Division (HEARD), EduAction, 2000. *Estimated Correlation Between HIV and School Enrolment.* Durban.
KwaZulu-Natal Department of Education and Culture. 2001. *Illness and Death Amongst Educators.* Durban.
National and Provincial Departments of Education. 2000. *Annual Schools Survey.* Pretoria.
Provincial Education Development Unit (PEDU), KwaZulu Natal Department of Education & Culture. 2001. *Future Estimates of Educators.* Durban.
Statistics South Africa. 1998. *The People of South Africa Population Census 1996.* Statistics South Africa, Pretoria.

CHAPTER 6

# Households

*Jeff Gow and Chris Desmond*

## Introduction

A comprehensive understanding of the extent to which the HIV/AIDS epidemic in South Africa will impact upon households has not been empirically investigated. Many predictions have been made as to how households might respond to the epidemic, especially in relation to increased medical costs for seriously ill household members, the additional burden of funeral expenses, and the growing number of orphans who need to be adopted by other households. What is known however is that the poor are most susceptible to these negative impacts, yet have the least resources to cope.

### Interaction of individuals and households

HIV infects the individual, but individuals rarely live in isolation. The illness and death of individuals impacts on the various institutions to which they belong. The household is one such institution and possibly the worst affected by the HIV/AIDS epidemic. The characteristics of the virus, its concentration in particular groups, the mode of transmission and progression, and the stigma attached to HIV/AIDS, result in the impacts at the household level being of particular concern.

In Africa the HIV/AIDS epidemic is concentrated in the most economically productive segment of the population (15–49 years old). The declining productivity of HIV-positive individuals is primarily and initially felt within the family. Deaths in this group lead to the loss of a productive household member, which results in loss of income and productive capacity as well as increased costs and changing expenditure patterns.

Foster (1996) identified three phases in the cycle of illness and death from AIDS:

1. the illness;
2. the death;
3. the longer-term aftermath.

Before analysing the impacts of each of these phases on households, it is worth noting the concentration of the epidemic in poorer communities as poverty plays a major role in determining a households susceptibility to infection and their vulnerability to the negative implications.

Cohen (1998) provided a conceptual economic analysis of the two-way relationship between HIV/AIDS and poverty. The poor are characterised by weak endowments of human (education, literacy) and financial resources, few marketable skills and generally poor health, all of which result in low productivity. These characteristics increase the risk of infection; an example is untreated sexually transmitted diseases (STDs) – a co-factor in the transmission of HIV. Inadequate access to health facilities in poor communities lead to higher numbers of STDs going untreated, facilitating the transmission of HIV. The situation that the poor find themselves in often prompts them to behave in ways which increase their chances of infection; migrant labour and sex work are examples. HIV infection, therefore, is concentrated in poor communities, and the effects of infections within them make them even poorer.

**Phase 1: Illness**

The concentration of HIV infection in the productive age-group has significant implications for the productive capacity and income of affected households.

During the illness phase, one of the first responses for those working in the informal sector is to move from directly productive activities into service-oriented jobs, (farming to selling goods) which are usually lower paid. This change allows the infected person to work when they can, as service jobs are generally less physically demanding. Income falls, and as the illness progresses the ability to work decreases, dragging income down further. A study in Côte d'Ivoire found that income in affected households was half that of the average household income (Bechu, 1998). This reduction in household income is often due not only to the loss of income associated with the ill member of the household, but also that with the diversion of activities of other members. For example, as HIV progresses to AIDS the level of care required increases, placing increased demands on other members of the household (Loewenson, 1998). Women are often given the added burden of having to care for the ill, in addition to the numerous household duties they typically perform, while possibly also being infected. Alternatively, children – particularly girls – are taken out of school to care for the sick or help with other household duties. If women are infected they require not only care, but also someone to take over their workload. Again children often have to fill this gap. If a male is infected his illness leaves a gap in the production process, which women or children are required to fill.

At the same time as income falls, costs increase, especially time, transport and medical costs. Health facilities are often located far from home and frequent journeys can be costly. The time involved in treatment places an added constraint on household labour. The medication required for the treatment is costly and requires re-balancing of the family budget (Bechu, 1998). In a Tanzanian study, it was found that people diagnosed with AIDS were more likely to seek medical attention than other terminally ill people, and were therefore more likely to incur out-of-pocket medical expenses (Ainsworth and Over, 1997). Moreover, household medical expenses tended to be much higher for AIDS than for other causes of death.

Expenditure patterns also change as a result of the illness. In the Côte d'Ivoire study it was found that the largest difference in household expenditure was spending on healthcare – which almost doubled (Bechu, 1998). The majority of this increase was for the benefit of the infected adult. Although total household expenditure on healthcare increased, the non-infected members received less than average because of the disproportionate amount used to care for the ill adult. The risk of illness and infection of other household members increased as a result of this disproportionate division. Over time the allocation to healthcare showed an increase as the illness progressed, and then spending fell in the closing stages. The fall was particularly marked for modern medicine; this was attributed to the disheartening effect of treatment that cannot cure. The increase in healthcare expenditure and the fall in income are accompanied by a fall in expenditure on basic needs. The shrinkage and re-allocation of the budget reduces food security within the home. The chances of malnutrition and sickness of other members are thereby increased. The weaker members within the household face greater risks. Children, in particular, occupy a weak bargaining position and therefore face the greatest risks. In the Côte d'Ivoire study two patterns in consumption were immediately evident. First, total consumption fell and later partially recovered. Second, basic needs, which include food, fell less than other categories of expenditure, and then almost fully recovered as families reduce other categories of expenditure to maintain consumption of necessities (Bechu, 1998).

The decreased income, increased costs and the ability of the household to cope with these changes has been linked to a number of household characteristics. In the Côte d'Ivoire study the fall in expenditure on basic needs was greater if the infected adult was female and the expenditure on health was greater if they were male (Bechu, 1998). Loewenson (1998) found that poor households incur greater costs than others, resulting from, *inter alia*, lack of social security cover and medical aid. Female death was associated with a stronger negative impact on consumption expenditure and average medical expenditure on terminally ill women was found to be less than the expenditure on men in the same condition. The level of education of the household head appeared to provide a degree of protection against the negative impacts of adult death. Further more the analysis suggested that the negative impacts of an AIDS death was greater than that of a non-AIDS death.

To summarise, the impact of HIV/AIDS illnesses at the household level is clearly serious. Household income falls while costs increase.

**Phase 2: Death**
The death of a prime-age adult is an obvious tragedy for any household. Survivors must contend not only with profound emotional loss, but also with medical and funeral expenses, plus the loss of income and services that a prime-age adult typically provides.

The economic impact of an AIDS death is larger on poorer households. Studies reveal that households experiencing an adult death draw on assets to cushion the shock of such an event. It follows that households with lower levels of assets will have more difficulty in coping with an adult death. Although studies indicate that households do employ coping mechanisms to overcome the prime-age adult deaths, they also show that households are generally worse off after the loss of a productive member. The impact of an adult death on poorer households is most starkly illustrated by changes in food expenditure and food consumption. For the poorest 50 per cent of households in the Tanzanian study, food expenditure dropped by nearly a third, while in the other 50 per cent of households, intake of both food produced at home and purchased food rose (Ainsworth and Over, 1997).

In most African countries a large funeral is an important statement. The transportation and feeding of guests and the cost of the coffin can drive families into debt and financial devastation (Foster, 1996). In the Tanzanian study, households that experienced a death had lower overall expenditures and devoted a larger share of their expenditure to funeral costs (Ainsworth and Over, 1997). It was also found that these households spent one-third less on items such as batteries, soap and clothing. Finally, in households that experienced a death, food produced by the household represented a larger share of consumption than in other households, while purchased food represented a smaller share. Evidence of the high cost of illness and death of an AIDS victim as compared to other deaths was found in a Ugandan study (Menon et al., 1998). It was found that while households that had not experienced an adult death in the period had increased ownership of durable goods and households that had experienced a non-AIDS death remained the same, those with AIDS deaths had suffered a decrease in ownership of these types of goods. Furthermore, livestock deaths and sale of draft power animals were higher and crop output lower in AIDS- death households. On average, households spent nearly 50 per cent more on funerals than they did on medical care.

Two broad observations can be made on the basis of these two studies: first, medical costs are only a portion of the cost of a prime-age adult death; and second, non-medical costs are likely to be similar regardless of the cause of death. Where these observations hold true, the direct impact of an AIDS death will not be much different from that of a non-AIDS death. Thus, the high costs to households from AIDS will usually be due to the large number of deaths caused by the epidemic, rather than by the fact that they are caused by AIDS.

## Phase 3: Longer-term adjustments
COPING STRATEGIES

A prime-age adult death has devastating impacts upon families and households. Survivors suffer economically, and the extent of this economic stress can be measured by the impact of an adult death on social indicators such as orphanhood, schooling, child nutrition and health, and poverty.

The economic shock of a prime-age adult death is mitigated to some extent by a variety of strategies that households use to cope. Survey data shows that when it comes to coping with the economic impact of such a loss, households are surprisingly resilient. Data on the mix of household coping strategies to the loss of an adult breadwinner come mostly from sub-Saharan Africa (Ainsworth and Over, 1998)

Four main coping strategies are observed:

1. doing nothing;
2. withdrawing savings or selling assets;
3. receiving assistance from other households;
4. altering household composition.

*Doing nothing*
Given the severe resource constraints facing many families and households which experience AIDS deaths, the capacity to respond in any meaningful way to overcome the difficulties now confronting the household, can sometimes be beyond their capabilities. In these circumstances, the most rational response can be to sit tight and change nothing about their living arrangements. If sufficient resources are still accessible then the immediate pressure to respond is absent.

*Dissaving and sale of assets*
The second coping mechanism of households is dissaving and sale of assets. Evidence from Tanzania and Uganda suggests that households draw down

savings or liquidate assets in response to a prime-age adult death. For example, radio ownership increased in households with no deaths and decreased in households that experienced death. In Tanzania, 51 per cent of the 80 households were members of savings and credit associations. After they experienced an adult death, participation had dropped to 36 per cent (Ainsworth and Over, 1998). Borrowing from microfinance organisations is also a common means of boosting the coping capacity of households. These bodies make loans to self-selecting groups, particularly women. In Zimbabwe, households were found to be selling land and cattle and taking children out of school to meet increased costs (Kwaramba, 1998). Although the sale of assets is a means of coping with the increased costs and reduced income, it has a series of negative implications for future economic potential. Similarly reductions in expenditure on basic needs and substituting cheaper, less nutritious food for the usual staples invariably introduced new problems. Nampanya-Serpell's (2000) study of 232 urban and 101 rural AIDS-affected families in Zambia found that there was a rapid transition from relative wealth to relative poverty in AIDS-affected families. This was particularly marked where a father died. Monthly disposable income of more than two-thirds of the families in this study fell by more than 80 per cent.

*Assistance from other households*
Help from neighbours and relatives is an important supplement to the efforts of households facing an adult death. In Tanzania, it was shown that 80 to 90 per cent of bereaved households were likely to receive assistance in cash or kind from other households. Focus group interviews in the sample villages found that besides the traditional savings and mutual assistance associations, residents of many villages had launched associations to help families affected by an AIDS death. Most of the associations were launched and operated by women, and many have regular meetings at which members make contributions in cash or kind (Liwuhla, 1998). It follows that households with lower levels of assets will experience greater difficulty in coping with the death of a prime-age adult than households with more assets. The coping strategies employed by households to adjust to the shock of a prime-age adult death hold many implications, particularly for the children of poor households.

*Altering household composition*
The most far reaching impact of an AIDS death within a family is the destruction of the family and household as a whole unit. Adult death tends to cluster in households, because of the nature of transmission of the virus. One or both adult parents dying has devastating effects on the capacity of households to remain intact. Where this is not possible, relatives and friends of the family take in individual children where the resources are available to

do so. Most commonly, grandparents – in particular, grandmothers – seem to take over this parenting role. The worst outcome for children is where no able-bodied adult is available to provide resources and maintain households and families together. This leads to destruction of the family unit as a household and displacement of children. In some fortuitous circumstances, sufficient resources are available for the children to maintain household structure despite the absence of any adults. These child-headed households face many difficulties in keeping their family together.

A Zimbabwean study of 215 households examined how adult deaths may cause the dissolution of households (Mutangadura, 2000). She found that about 40 per cent of the sample households had taken in orphans who had lost both parents. Sixty five per cent of households where the deceased adult female used to live before her death were reported to be no longer in existence in both the urban and rural sites. This lends weight to the supposition that often the worst impact is invisible because it is among those who are not counted.

In order to respond most effectively to this crisis with the limited resources available, information is needed, firstly to understand the rate at which households are affected by HIV/AIDS, and secondly what coping mechanisms individual households adopt in response to the epidemic's economic impact. To this end a survey of selected households in the Bergville district, KwaZulu-Natal, was undertaken. The overall objective of the survey was to investigate the impacts of serious illness and the presence of orphans on households in the Bergville community.

**Data collection and sources**
The method which was used was in-depth surveys of a selected number of households who have either a seriously ill member, an orphan, or were not currently affected by the epidemic at all. These households were selected by local enumerators on the basis of their knowledge of the presence or otherwise of people with these above characteristics in the households.

The sampling frame consisted of all of the households that belonged to the Amazizi and Amangwane Tribal Authorities, as well as wards from the 11 Settlements. The individual communities in the Bergville area that were surveyed were: Ukhombe, Zwelisha, Emamfemfetheni, Rooihoek and Hoffental. A household scan was conducted and every third household was asked to respond to a one-page questionnaire on household structure, illness and orphans. Based on this scan households were divided into three categories:

1. households that contained children whose mother was not alive (orphan);
2. households with an adult aged 15–49 who had been so ill in the last two weeks that they were not able to attend work for more than five days or were bed ridden (illness);

3. households where neither of those two types of people were present (control).

Three groups of approximately 60 households each were selected. In early 2001, 178 households were surveyed.

The following were conditions for undertaking the survey:

- Households had already been identified, approached and agreed to participate in the survey.
- Two key informants per household were available to be interviewed (this was necessary as usually the people in charge of spending the money were not the people who earned the money).
- Identified households were in not more than 15 walking distance clusters i.e. 12 households from each cluster, with a mixture of different types of households.
- The fieldwork took place over weekends to make sure that all key informants were at home. Households had members who were migrant workers who only came home monthly so it was necessary to schedule interviews to capture those people.

**Limitations**

The primary limitation of the survey is that it is not clear how good a proxy adult illness is for HIV illness. It was assumed to be close; given that in 1999 prevalence among women attending antenatal clinics in the area was already over 21 per cent. HIV should be accounting for a high proportion of adult illness.

Secondly, some households when revisited no longer belonged in their original group. For example, some households were found not to have orphans. They had said they did, believing that some assistance might follow. Other households no longer contained adults who were ill. Households that had changed group were re-classified on data capture to the correct group. This is what accounts for the slightly uneven split between the groups.

Finally, the survey suffers the same limitation as any other cross-sectional assessment of impact. Unless it can be assumed that prior to the impact of illness, HIV-affected households had similar characteristics to a random sample of non-infected households the survey cannot measure impact.

## *Demographics and general household characteristics*

The detailed data in this section show the characteristics of the surveyed households. Households were divided up into three types: orphan, illness and control.

## Household structure

The three types of household had average household numbers of nine. More females were present in all three types of household though not by significant numbers. Orphan households were more likely to be headed by a female (57 per cent) than illness households (47 per cent) or control households (42 per cent). The high proportion of retired persons in orphan households again suggests orphans staying with their grandparents and, based on the gender breakdown, they are staying with their grandmother. Examination of the marital status of adults also shows a higher proportion of widows/widowers within orphan households: ten per cent compared to six per cent (illness) and seven per cent (control). No households in the sample were headed by anyone below the age of 20 years.

The results of the marital status variable also began to raise the question of mobility and migrants. In both the orphan and the illness households the majority of married couples were not living together. The average age of household members across all three types of household was 23 years. Just over one-third of household members were actively engaged in economic activity. The remaining two-thirds of household members were either children under five years, attending school, retired people or housewives. There were no gender differences between males and females in engaging in economic activity.

Table 6.1 Number of households, by household status.

| Orphan | 63 |
| Illness | 59 |
| Control | 56 |
| **Total** | **178** |

Table 6.2 The gender breakdown of household members by status and total.

|  | Orphan | Illness | Control | Total |
| --- | --- | --- | --- | --- |
| Male | 283 | 256 | 239 | 778 |
| Female | 303 | 275 | 294 | 872 |
| **Total** | **586** | **531** | **533** | **1 650** |
| **Average household size** | 9.4 | 9.0 | 9.4 | 9.3 |

**Table 6.3  Breakdown by gender of household heads.**

|  | Orphan | Illness | Control | Total |
|---|---|---|---|---|
| Male | 27 | 30 | 32 | 89 |
| Female | 36 | 27 | 24 | 87 |
| **Total** | **63** | **57** | **56** | **178** |

**Table 6.4  Average age of household heads.**

|  | Percentage female head | Average age of household head |
|---|---|---|
| Orphans | 57 | 59 |
| Illness | 47 | 52 |
| Control | 42 | 54 |
| **Total** | **49** | **55** |

**Table 6.5  Vocation of all members by household status.**

|  | Orphan | Illness | Control | Total |
|---|---|---|---|---|
| Baby, pre-school or crèche | 88 | 84 | 91 | 263 |
| Scholar/student | 238 | 184 | 198 | 620 |
| School-going age – not attending | 11 | 20 | 14 | 45 |
| Retired | 38 | 26 | 23 | 87 |
| Disabled – not seeking work | 6 | 10 | 4 | 20 |
| Housewife/unpaid work | 16 | 20 | 23 | 59 |
| Unemployed – seeking work | 77 | 90 | 82 | 249 |
| Unemployed – not seeking work | 18 | 20 | 24 | 62 |
| Employed full time | 29 | 23 | 30 | 82 |
| Employed part time | 48 | 30 | 33 | 111 |
| Self employed | 17 | 24 | 11 | 52 |
| **Total** | **586** | **531** | **533** | **1 650** |

## Mobility

Over 22 per cent of members of the households spent more than half of the previous month absent from the household. There was no difference between males and females in absences. Movement out of the households mainly occurred for employment opportunities (46 per cent). The second most common reason for leaving was to be looked after by other distant family members (20 per cent). Females were more likely to move away from the household than were males. More members of the illness and control households moved away than from orphan households. Over 50 per cent of people in both households moved away for employment opportunities.

Table 6.6  Death or departure from household by gender of the deceased/departed in the past 12 months.

|  | Male | Female | Total |
|---|---|---|---|
| Dead | 24 | 48 | 72 |
| Moved/left | 46 | 58 | 104 |
| **Total** | **70** | **106** | **176** |

Table 6.7  Reasons for member of household departing, by gender.

|  | Male | Female | Total |
|---|---|---|---|
| To be looked after by other family members | 10 | 12 | 22 |
| To help other family members | 2 | 5 | 7 |
| Schooling/study opportunities | 0 | 2 | 2 |
| Job opportunities | 28 | 20 | 47 |
| Married/went to live with partner | 3 | 11 | 14 |
| Ran away | 2 | 2 | 4 |
| To have own home/place | 1 | 5 | 6 |
| Moved with parents | 0 | 1 | 1 |
| **Total** | **46** | **58** | **104** |

**Table 6.8 Reason for departure by household status.**

|  | Orphan | Illness | Control | Total |
|---|---|---|---|---|
| To be looked after by other family members | 9 | 3 | 7 | 22 |
| To help other family members | 4 | 2 | 1 | 7 |
| Schooling/study opportunities | 1 | 0 | 1 | 2 |
| Job opportunities | 7 | 20 | 21 | 48 |
| Married/went to live with partner | 6 | 5 | 3 | 14 |
| Ran away | 2 | 1 | 1 | 4 |
| To have own home/place | 0 | 6 | 0 | 6 |
| Moved with parents | 0 | 0 | 1 | 1 |
| **Total** | **29** | **37** | **38** | **104** |

**Illness**

Over seven per cent of all household members were ill for more than five days in the previous three months. The most common illness reported was chest infection (22 per cent), followed by headaches and other pain (ten per cent each). Not surprisingly, the majority of reported illness came from illness households with over 50 per cent. Orphan households had higher levels of reported illness (27 per cent) than control households (20 per cent).

Primary caregivers were household heads in 42 per cent of cases. Children were the primary caregiver in 25 per cent of instances. Traditional healthcare services were accessed in over ten per cent of episodes. Western doctors and clinics were more commonly used, with transport to and from all forms of care being a significant factor here. In over 16 per cent of episodes no treatment was sought or forthcoming.

**Table 6.9 Adults sick/bedridden for more than five days in the last three months.**

|  | Yes | No | Total |
|---|---|---|---|
| **Total** | 119 | 1 531 | 1 650 |

**Table 6.10 The primary caregiver.**

|  | Orphan | Illness | Control | Total |
|---|---|---|---|---|
| Household head | 16 | 26 | 9 | 51 |
| Other adult | 7 | 15 | 4 | 26 |
| Children | 7 | 13 | 10 | 30 |
| Family member from outside | 0 | 1 | 0 | 1 |
| Neighbour | 3 | 1 | 0 | 4 |
| No-one | 0 | 5 | 0 | 5 |
| Do not know | 0 | 1 | 1 | 2 |
| **Total** | **33** | **62** | **24** | **119** |

## Death

Over four per cent of the members of the surveyed households had died in the previous 12 months. Not surprisingly, orphan households had experienced the highest level of death accounting for 57 per cent of reported deaths. This corresponded to seven per cent of orphan household members. Illness and control households had experienced the same level of absolute deaths. In percentage terms these were both three per cent of household members. A wide variety of illnesses were reported as the cases of death. Significantly, AIDS was only mentioned once out of 72 deaths.

**Table 6.11 Death or departure from household in the past 12 months.**

|  | Death | Moved | Total |
|---|---|---|---|
| Orphans | 41 | 29 | 70 |
| Illness | 16 | 37 | 53 |
| Control | 15 | 38 | 53 |
| **Total** | **72** | **104** | **176** |

## Orphans and other children

Eighty per cent of children lived with either their natural mother or father. Twenty-seven children were identified as orphans where both parents had died. Deceased mothers were more likely to have been both the primary caregiver and financial provider to the orphans than were deceased fathers. Fathers and mothers of orphans had died in equal numbers. A pattern of recent death of natural parents was emerging with over half of these parents having died in the preceding three years. The primary caregivers to these children in two-thirds of the cases were the child's grandparents, especially the grandmother.

After the death of their mother, many children become members of their grandmother's household; this is even more marked when both parents have died. The reliance on grandparents to provide care after the death of parents is dangerous and will become increasingly so as the epidemic progresses. When the grandparents die these children face being orphaned again. The question of who will care for them then remains unanswered. Furthermore, grandparents generally rely on government pensions. Although this represents a stable income, it is fixed and they have little opportunities to increase it. They, therefore, may be able to cope with a few orphans, but as numbers increase and income does not, their ability to meet the financial costs of care will be strained. The grandparents of the future are dying in the present. Who will care for the children in 15 years time?

Table 6.12 Which parent(s) all children live with.

|  | Yes | No | Total |
|---|---|---|---|
| Natural mother | 391 | 52 | 443 |
| Natural father | 266 | 123 | 389 |
| **Total** | **657** | **175** | **832** |

Table 6.13 Relationship to the head of household of children under the age of 16 who have lost both parents in households with orphan status.

|  | Frequency |
|---|---|
| Son/daughter | 1 |
| Grandchild | 15 |
| Brother/sister | 2 |
| Niece/nephew | 4 |
| Other relative | 5 |
| **Total** | **27** |

**Table 6.14** Relationship to the head of orphan households of children under the age of 16 who have lost their mother.

|  | Frequency |
|---|---|
| Son/daughter | 14 |
| Adopted/foster child | 1 |
| Grandchild | 59 |
| Brother/sister | 2 |
| Niece/nephew | 9 |
| Other relative | 5 |
| **Total** | **90** |

**Table 6.15** Relationship to the head of orphan households of children under the age of 16 who have lost their mother but not their father.

|  | Orphan | Illness | Control | Total |
|---|---|---|---|---|
| Son/daughter | 13 | 0 | 0 | 13 |
| Adopted foster/child | 1 | 0 | 0 | 1 |
| Grandchild | 42 | 2 | 2 | 46 |
| Niece/nephew | 3 | 0 | 0 | 3 |
| **Total** | **59** | **2** | **2** | **63** |

**Table 6.16** Parental loss for all households by gender.

|  | Frequency |
|---|---|
| Mother | 100 |
| Father | 104 |
| **Total** | **204** |

**Table 6.17  Number of years since parents death.**

|  | Frequency |
|---|---|
| 1 | 29 |
| 2 | 38 |
| 3 | 35 |
| 4 | 16 |
| 5 | 14 |
| 6 | 9 |
| 7 | 9 |
| 8 | 4 |
| 9 | 6 |
| 10 | 1 |
| More than 10 | 11 |
| Do not know | 2 |
| **Total** | **174** |

**Table 6.18  Parents who were the financial provider to the child prior to their death, by gender.**

|  | Mother | Father | Total |
|---|---|---|---|
| Yes | 92 | 66 | 158 |
| No | 8 | 35 | 43 |
| Do not know | 0 | 3 | 3 |
| **Total** | **100** | **104** | **204** |

**Table 6.19  Parents who were the primary caregiver prior to death, by gender.**

|  | Mother | Father | Total |
|---|---|---|---|
| Yes | 95 | 58 | 153 |
| No | 5 | 46 | 51 |
| **Total** | **100** | **104** | **204** |

## Education

School fees played a significant role in approximately one-third of cases where children did not attend school. Absenteeism from school ran at about seven per cent of students. Forty-five per cent of those who had attended school had only obtained a primary school education with only 14 per cent having completed school up to the last two years of high school. Very few household members had completed a post school education qualification (2.5 per cent).

Table 6.20 Reason for not attending school of children who don't attend school.

|  | Orphan | Illness | Control | Frequency |
|---|---|---|---|---|
| Could not pay school fees | 3 | 5 | 8 | 16 |
| Too ill to attend | 1 | 5 | 0 | 6 |
| Looking after own child | 1 | 2 | 1 | 4 |
| Fell pregnant | 1 | 1 | 2 | 4 |
| No reason | 0 | 1 | 1 | 2 |
| Told that child too young to go to school | 2 | 1 | 0 | 3 |
| Mother died, moved to the area – no place | 1 | 0 | 0 | 1 |
| Application refused – no birth certificate | 1 | 0 | 1 | 2 |
| Ran away from school | 0 | 1 | 0 | 1 |
| Dropped out | 0 | 0 | 1 | 1 |
| Poor performance at school | 0 | 2 | 0 | 2 |
| Disabled | 1 | 2 | 0 | 3 |
| **Total** | **11** | **20** | **14** | **45** |

Table 6.21 Highest school education completed.

|  | Orphan | Illness | Control | Total |
|---|---|---|---|---|
| Grade 1 | 27 | 30 | 27 | 59 |
| Grade 2 | 33 | 27 | 28 | 88 |
| Grade 3 | 36 | 26 | 38 | 100 |
| Grade 4 | 39 | 34 | 31 | 104 |
| Grade 5 | 35 | 24 | 37 | 96 |
| Grade 6 | 33 | 43 | 29 | 105 |
| Grade 7 | 53 | 40 | 32 | 125 |
| Grade 8 | 33 | 42 | 35 | 110 |
| Grade 9 | 30 | 21 | 28 | 79 |
| Grade 10 | 38 | 26 | 31 | 95 |
| Grade 11 | 27 | 32 | 28 | 87 |
| Grade 12 | 33 | 25 | 30 | 88 |
| Disabled schooling | 0 | 2 | 0 | 2 |
| **Total** | **434** | **391** | **397** | **1 222** |

## 128  Impacts and Interventions

**Table 6.22  Highest post-school education/qualification.**

|  | Orphan | Illness | Control | Total |
|---|---|---|---|---|
| Technikon diploma | 0 | 3 | 2 | 5 |
| Other diploma | 1 | 1 | 0 | 2 |
| Certificate | 7 | 11 | 7 | 25 |
| None | 426 | 376 | 388 | 1 190 |
| **Total** | **434** | **391** | **397** | **1 222** |

## *Services and facilities available to households*

Even before considering the impact of adult illness and death, and orphaning, it is essential to note the existing poverty and violations of children's rights. The data in this section shows that most households have access to few resources beyond the most basic needed to survive.

### Physical resources

HOUSING

The vast majority of households (over 90 per cent) lived in traditional house structures made with traditional materials like mud, brick and dung. Less than ten per cent of households had a permanent house in the brick and block style. A few of the remaining households lived in shacks made from plastic, cardboard and/or corrugated iron. The size of the household required many rooms to accommodate members. The most common number of rooms for a household was five, six or seven.

WATER SUPPLIES

Only one out of 178 households had piped internal water in the homestead. Only 71 out of 178 had access to clean, piped and government supplied water. The remaining 107 households had to access water from wells or boreholes, dams, flowing streams or springs located away from the household. There were no significant differences in water supply sources across the three different types of households. Almost half of all households relied upon rainwater for irrigating gardens.

SANITATION

No house had a flushing water-based toilet. Fifteen per cent of households did not have a toilet attached to the homestead at all, whilst the other 85 per cent of households used pit toilets without water and frequently without ventilation. Refuse disposal took place at home with approximately half of households burying it and the rest burning it on site.

CONSUMER GOODS
One-sixth of households had cellular phones, there being no significant difference in their distribution among the three types of household. Radio ownership was widespread with over 70 per cent of households having access. Televisions were owned by a much smaller number of households with less than 30 per cent being connected. Fridges (of any description) were present in only ten per cent of households. Motor car ownership was even less common with only 14 out of 178 households having a motor car.

UTILITIES
Only one-third of households were connected to electricity and only one-third of those households used electricity for cooking. The main energy source used for cooking was wood, which was employed by almost two-thirds of households. The other significant source of cooking energy was paraffin. Heating is an issue in the Bergville area in winter and over 80 per cent used wood as the main heating source.

**Financial resources**
MEDICAL AID
Very few households had access to medical aid, only six out of 178 households. With no orphan household having medical aid at all.

SAVINGS AND BORROWINGS
Only 39 bank savings accounts were held by the 1 650 people in the 178 households. These were shared equally between males and females. Stokvels or community savings groups were held by 24 out of 178 households with females being the instigator in 22 out of 24 of those households. With little individual or household interaction with banks it is not surprising that the number of cash loans held by members of all households were very low. More commonly, credit was obtained directly when purchasing consumer goods with approximately 20 per cent of households having hire purchase commitments. Informal credit arrangements were a source of borrowing for about ten per cent of households.

## *Income*
Incomes of all households in the sample were relatively low. Given the large average household size this translates into relatively few resources being available on a per capita basis.

**Income sources**
Of the 1 650 individuals in the sample households, 369 individual income earners were identified with 15 of those earning income from two sources.

Twenty-two per cent of the members of all sampled households were earning income. This from an economically active group of 33 per cent of individuals in the sample.

Employment, whether formal or informal made up 50 per cent of income sources for members of all households earning income. The informal sector contributing 32 per cent and the formal sector 18 per cent which reflects the lack of economic activity in the Bergville district and the high levels of unemployment. Self-employment was a significant source of income with 17 per cent earning their own income. Pensions were also a source of income for 18 per cent of the income earners. This mainly reflects the large number of grandmothers in the community.

The number of income earners in orphan households was surprisingly more than the number in illness or control households. Closer examination showed that a greater variety of members in the orphan households earned income compared with the illness and control households. The first four earners were in the vast majority of cases adults. These other earners are youths or children who, because of the existence of orphans in the household and hence the greater demand on resources, need to contribute. The first four earners for illness households contributed 90 per cent of income compared to 79 per cent in the control households and only 75 per cent in orphan households.

Table 6.23  Income sources.

|  | Orphan | Illness | Control | Total |
|---|---|---|---|---|
| Formal sector employment | 23 | 22 | 25 | 70 |
| Informal sector employment | 48 | 31 | 44 | 123 |
| Operating their own stall | 14 | 19 | 11 | 44 |
| Operating their own farm | 1 | 3 | 0 | 4 |
| Selling agricultural produce | 4 | 3 | 1 | 8 |
| Growing or selling dagga | 1 | 3 | 8 | 12 |
| Remittances | 2 | 3 | 3 | 8 |
| Government old age pension | 30 | 22 | 15 | 67 |
| Pension from work | 1 | 5 | 0 | 6 |
| Unemployment insurance fund | 1 | 1 | 0 | 2 |
| Worker's compensation | 2 | 0 | 0 | 2 |
| Any type of grant (under 18) | 2 | 4 | 2 | 8 |
| Any type of grant (18 years & over) | 5 | 2 | 0 | 7 |
| Stokvel | 3 | 0 | 0 | 3 |
| Lobola/dowry | 1 | 0 | 0 | 1 |
| Family not resident income | 6 | 5 | 4 | 15 |
| Scholarships and bursaries | 0 | 0 | 3 | 3 |
| Other financial assistance | 0 | 0 | 1 | 1 |
| **Total** | 144 | 122 | 118 | 384 |

**Personal and household income**
Individual incomes earned by members of orphan and illness households were significantly higher (approximately 20 per cent) than those earned by members from control households. This trend was exacerbated when account was taken at the household level where average incomes in orphan and illness households were 30 per cent higher than control households. Therefore, there are substantial differences in per capita incomes also.

A similar story emerges when the gender of the household head is considered. Female-headed households on average received 25 per cent less income per month than male-headed households. Even when these incomes are controlled for the influence of pensions the differential is still 20 per cent in favour of male-headed households.

Both orphan and illness households reported incomes greater than the control group. There are a number of possible explanations for this. Households with greater status in the community may be more prone to infection as members have greater access to sex. Income in these households may fall following illness, but may have been much higher to begin with. Households with greater income may also be more prepared to absorb orphans. The orphan households appear to have more income earners. Income in orphan households is bolstered by the presence of older members who obtain government pensions, in addition to the earnings of working adult members.

Although the impact of illness is unclear, the impact of death is unambiguous. The impact of a recent death on all types of households is apparent. The mean household income across the sample was R1 330 for those who had not experienced a death in the last 12 months and R848 for those who had. That is, incomes in households that had experienced a death in the previous twelve months were 56 per cent less than those that had not experienced the tragedy of the loss of a family member. Funeral costs represented, on average, twice the monthly income of the household. Not surprisingly the majority of funerals in the sample had been paid for by orphan households, over 50 per cent of whom had suffered a death of a household member in the previous 12 months, compared to 25 per cent of illness households and 21 per cent of control households. In response to such an impact, households had adopted a number of strategies. Such responses raise a number of concerns. The sale of assets, particularly if they are productive, has long-term implications for the wellbeing of the household. Borrowing money from family, friends or stokvels, although possible now, may become increasingly difficult as AIDS deaths escalate.

**Table 6.24  Individual household and per capita mean monthly.**

|         | Individual earner mean (n = 369) | Household mean | Household per capita mean |
|---------|---|---|---|
| Orphan  | 597 | 1 328 | 142 |
| Illness | 612 | 1 366 | 168 |
| Control | 485 | 1 009 | 117 |
| **Total** | **567** | **1 240** | **143** |

**Table 6.25  Total household income by gender of household head per month.**

|        | Mean |
|--------|------|
| Male   | 1 314 |
| Female | 1 056 |
| **Total** | **1 111** |

**Table 6.26  Total household income by gender of household head, excluding pensions, per month.**

|        | Mean |
|--------|------|
| Male   | 1 225 |
| Female | 996 |
| **Total** | **1 066** |

**Table 6.27  Total household income of households who have experienced a recent death (in the past 12 months) compared to non-death households, per month.**

|          | Mean |
|----------|------|
| No death | 1 330 |
| Death    | 848 |

## *Expenditure and consumption*
Consumption in all of the households is constrained by two major factors: comparatively small household income and large household size, both of which increase dependency ratios.

With small incomes available to households (approximately R1 000 per month) expenditure was targeted toward essential items like food, housing, transport and education.

### Food expenditure
Between 37 and 40 per cent of expenditure across all three types of household went on food. A large percentage of food expenditure went on storable items (dried or canned), which is understandable in the absence of wide ownership of fridges. Meat products were significant, accounting for over 15 per cent of food expenditure.

### Non-food expenditure
Around 35 per cent of total household expenditure went on regular non-food items like loan repayments, transport, entertainment and utilities. Occasional non-food expenditure on items such as education, insurance, and cultural activities (for example weddings, marriages and the payment of labola) contributed around ten to 18 per cent of household expenditure. Whilst these cultural activities are infrequent they are major expenses at the time of occurrence. Orphan and control household spent 18 per cent of total expenditure on occasional non-food items whilst orphan households only spent ten per cent of total expenditure on these types of items.

### Healthcare expenditure
This was uniformly low across all types of households. Given the level of illness in the wider Bergville community this was surprising with healthcare expenditure ranging from one per cent in control households to two per cent in orphan households and three per cent in illness households.

### Credit repayment expenditure
This varied significantly by household type. Illness households committed ten per cent of total expenditure to debt reduction, whilst only five per cent of expenditure by orphan households and seven per cent of expenditure by control households went on debt reduction.

**Table 6.28** Frequency of occasional non-food expenditure (all households which reported).

|  | Orphan | Illness | Control | Total |
|---|---|---|---|---|
| Holidays | 2 | 3 | 4 | 9 |
| Jewellery, watches | 1 | 1 | 0 | 2 |
| Ceremonies (weddings) | 6 | 3 | 10 | 19 |
| Labola | 2 | 2 | 2 | 6 |
| Funerals | 16 | 8 | 10 | 34 |
| School fees & tuition | 58 | 55 | 52 | 165 |
| Books and uniforms | 41 | 42 | 38 | 121 |
| Crèche/childcare | 2 | 3 | 4 | 9 |
| Other school expenses | 21 | 13 | 17 | 51 |
| Life insurance, funeral policies | 26 | 20 | 22 | 68 |
| Medical aid | 0 | 1 | 2 | 3 |
| Special security door | 0 | 0 | 1 | 1 |
| Purchasing dogs for security | 0 | 1 | 0 | 1 |
| Vehicle purchase | 0 | 2 | 0 | 2 |
| None | 2 | 3 | 4 | 9 |
| **Total** | **177** | **157** | **166** | **500** |

**Table 6.29** Value of occasional non-food expenditure (Rands in the past 12 months).

|  | Mean |
|---|---|
| Holidays | 280 |
| Jewellery, watches | 430 |
| Ceremonies (weddings) | 2 775 |
| Labola | 7 366 |
| Funerals | 2 713 |
| School fees & tuition | 219 |
| Books and uniforms | 232 |
| Crèche/childcare | 40 |
| Other school expenses | 52 |
| Life insurance, funeral policies | 73 |
| Medical aid | 226 |
| Special security door | 200 |
| Purchasing dogs for security | 10 |
| Vehicle purchase | 6 750 |

Table 6.30 Expenditure on different forms of healthcare (Rands in the past 12 months).

|  | Frequency | Mean |
|---|---|---|
| Doctors | 71 | 190 |
| Hospital/Clinic | 56 | 74 |
| Medical supplies | 5 | 93 |
| Transport to and from the hospital/clinic | 86 | 55 |
| Transport to and from traditional healers | 21 | 78 |
| Traditional healers fees | 27 | 366 |
| Traditional medicine | 15 | 151 |
| None | 56 | 0 |
| **Total** | **337** | **130** |

Table 6.31 Value of healthcare expenditure.

|  | Orphan | Illness | Control | Average |
|---|---|---|---|---|
| Frequency | 90 | 123 | 68 |  |
| **Mean** | **137** | **148** | **87** | **130** |

## Total Expenditure (Rands per month)

Table 6.32 Average household monthly expenditure.

| Expenditures | Orphan | Illness | Control | Average |
|---|---|---|---|---|
| Food | 323 | 390 | 303 | 339 |
| Regular non-food | 330 | 346 | 282 | 319 |
| Occasional non-food | 148 | 97 | 147 | 131 |
| Healthcare | 17 | 26 | 9 | 17 |
| HP and informal credit | 51 | 94 | 57 | 67 |
| **Total** | **869** | **953** | **798** | **873** |

## Adverse events and coping strategies employed
The extent of adverse events and the coping strategies employed by the different types of households over the preceding twelve months are discussed in this section.

### Death
Looking at the most serious issue first, death, it is not surprising that orphan households have experienced the highest level of death in the previous 12 months. Over half of orphan households had experienced the trauma of a death during that time compared with a quarter of illness households and a fifth of control households. Using any reckoning the level of death experienced in all of these households is very high. If these households are representative of the wider community this would seem to indicate that the level of death in the Bergville region is extraordinarily high.

The coping strategies that were employed in the three types of household to the death of a household member varied significantly. The most common strategy in orphan households was to do nothing. This approach accounted for about one-third of household responses. Approximately one-fifth of orphan households either sold assets or used savings or borrowed money from family or friends to cope. Only one-tenth of households borrowed money from a money-lender.

The most common strategy of illness households was to borrow money from family or friends. This approach accounted for over one-half of household responses. Other strategies employed included selling assets or using savings, borrowing money from a money-lender or stokvel. One household received support from an employer and one household chose to do nothing.

The most common strategy of control households was to borrow money from family or friends. This approach accounted for almost one-half of household responses. Other strategies employed included selling assets or using savings, and borrowing money from a money-lender. One household received support from an employer and two households chose to do nothing.

### Occurrences in the previous 12 months

Table 6.33  Death of a household member or other family member.

|  | Orphan | Illness | Control | Total |
|---|---|---|---|---|
| Yes | 32 | 15 | 12 | 59 |
| No | 30 | 44 | 45 | 119 |
| **Total** | **62** | **59** | **57** | **178** |

**Table 6.34  Death: Financial coping strategy.**

|  | Orphan | Illness | Control | Total |
|---|---|---|---|---|
| Sell assets or use savings | 6 | 1 | 3 | 10 |
| Borrow money from money lender | 3 | 2 | 1 | 6 |
| Borrow money from family or friends | 7 | 8 | 5 | 20 |
| Borrow money from stokvel | 1 | 2 | 0 | 3 |
| Get non-financial help from others | 1 | 0 | 0 | 1 |
| Use insurance/medical aid | 2 | 0 | 0 | 2 |
| Financial support from employer | 1 | 1 | 1 | 3 |
| Do nothing | 11 | 1 | 2 | 14 |
| **Total** | **32** | **15** | **12** | **59** |

## Serious illness or injury

Not surprisingly, illness households experienced the highest level of serious illness or injury in the three types of household. Approximately two-thirds of them had experienced serious illness or injury in the previous 12 months. Almost one-third and one-quarter of orphan and control household respectively had a household member who had experienced serious illness or injury in the previous 12 months.

The coping strategies that were employed in the three types of household to the serious illness or injury of a household member did not vary significantly. The most common strategy in illness households was to borrow money from family or friends. This approach accounted for approximately two-thirds of these households responses. Other significant responses included selling assets or using savings, and borrowing money from a money-lender. One household received support from an employer and six households chose to do nothing.

The most common strategy in orphan households was to borrow money from family or friends. This approach accounted for almost one-half of these households responses. Other significant responses included selling assets or using savings, borrowing money from a money-lender or using insurance or medical aid. Six households chose to do nothing.

The most common strategy in control households was to borrow money from family or friends. This approach accounted for over one-half of these households responses. Other significant responses included selling assets or using savings, or doing nothing.

**Table 6.35 Serious illness or injury of a household member.**

|  | Orphan | Illness | Control | Total |
|---|---|---|---|---|
| Yes | 19 | 34 | 16 | 69 |
| No | 43 | 25 | 41 | 109 |
| **Total** | **62** | **59** | **57** | **178** |

**Table 6.36 Serious illness or injury: Financial coping strategy.**

| Status | Orphan | Illness | Control | Total |
|---|---|---|---|---|
| Sell assets or use savings | 3 | 4 | 2 | 9 |
| Borrow money from money lender | 1 | 2 | 0 | 3 |
| Borrow money from family or friends | 8 | 21 | 9 | 38 |
| Use insurance/medical aid | 1 | 0 | 0 | 1 |
| Financial support from employer | 0 | 1 | 0 | 1 |
| Do nothing | 6 | 6 | 5 | 17 |
| **Total** | **19** | **34** | **16** | **69** |

**Loss of regular job**

The loss of a regular job by a household member has significant income effects for all types of households given the high level of unemployment in the Bergville region, the high dependency ratios and large average household size. Approximately one-sixth of all three types of household experienced the loss of a regular job and therefore income by a household member over the previous 12 months.

All three types of household did nothing as the most common response. This reflects the lack of opportunity for alternative jobs in the community as well as the limited resources at hand. Reduced consumption by household members would inevitably result.

In the orphan households doing nothing accounted for over half of household responses. Other significant responses included selling assets or taking children out of school. This latter response is particularly worrying given the likelihood of that child not returning to school whilst the household continues to suffer financial stress as a result of loss of income.

In the illness household the only other response was to sell assets or use savings. In the control households other significant responses were to borrow money from a money-lender or stokvel or send someone away from the household.

**Cut off or decrease in remittances**
At least two of each of the three types of household experienced total or partial decrease in remittances from family members away from Bergville. The coping strategies employed mainly involved reducing consumption, although one control household did borrow money from a money-lender.

**Abandonment or divorce**
Only one household from the illness households reported abandonment or divorce. The response of this household was to do nothing.

**Theft, fire or destruction of property**
Four orphan and three illness households had experienced theft, fire or destruction of household property. The four orphan households did not employ any coping mechanisms. Two of the three illness households borrowed money from family or friends.

**Loss of crops or livestock**
Six orphan households, three illness and five control households experienced loss of crops or livestock. The majority response was to do nothing. This was employed in ten out of 14 households. Of the remaining four households, two households sold assets or used savings, one borrowed money from a money lender and one borrowed money from family or friends.

**Failure or bankruptcy of business**
All three types of household reported at least one failure or bankruptcy from operating their own businesses. The response of two of these households was to do nothing whilst the other household got non-financial help from others.

Table 6.37  **Loss of a regular job of a household member.**

|  | Orphan | Illness | Control | Total |
|---|---|---|---|---|
| Yes | 11 | 11 | 11 | 33 |
| No | 51 | 48 | 46 | 145 |
| **Total** | **62** | **59** | **57** | **178** |

**Table 6.38  Loss of regular job: Financial coping strategy.**

|  | Orphan | Illness | Control | Total |
|---|---|---|---|---|
| Sell assets or use savings | 3 | 2 | 0 | 5 |
| Borrow money from money lender | 0 | 0 | 1 | 1 |
| Borrow money from stokvel | 0 | 0 | 1 | 1 |
| Take children out of school | 2 | 0 | 0 | 2 |
| Send someone away | 0 | 0 | 1 | 1 |
| Do nothing | 6 | 9 | 8 | 23 |
| **Total** | **11** | **11** | **11** | **33** |

## Time use patterns

The time use patterns of the different types of households are represented as hours spent per day in various activities as reported by the head of the household or the person interviewed who represented the household.

The orphan and illness households spent more time on personal care (including medical care), cooking, cleaning and food preparation, fetching water and firewood, and home maintenance and yard work than did the control households. On average these totalled approximately half an hour more on each of the three tasks for the orphan and illness household than the control households.

No significant time differences were experienced between the three types of household in the time spent on sleeping, child care, care of the sick, shopping, subsistence production, wage work or looking for work. Interestingly, time spent on care of the sick did not vary significantly between the three types of households.

The extra workload for orphan and illness households resulted in less leisure time being available to them. Orphan households had on average four-and-a-half leisure hours, control households five-and-a-half and illness households three leisure hours per day. This indicates the extra time pressure that the orphan and illness households experience as the result of having an orphan or seriously ill person present in their midsts.

## Time spent on various life activities (in hours per day)

**Table 6.39  Personal care: Dressing, eating, and receiving medical care.**

|  | Mean |
|---|---|
| Orphan | 2.1 |
| Illness | 2.2 |
| Control | 1.6 |
| **Average** | **1.9** |

### Table 6.40  Cooking, cleaning, washing clothes, food preparation.

|  | Mean |
|---|---|
| Orphan | 3.6 |
| Illness | 3.7 |
| Control | 3.3 |
| **Average** | **3.5** |

### Table 6.41  Fetching water and/or firewood/dung.

|  | Mean |
|---|---|
| Orphan | 0.8 |
| Illness | 1.3 |
| Control | 1.0 |
| **Average** | **1.0** |

### Table 6.42  Home construction and maintenance, yard work.

|  | Mean |
|---|---|
| Orphan | 1.4 |
| Illness | 1.2 |
| Control | 1.0 |
| **Average** | **1.2** |

### Table 6.43  Attending school.

|  | Mean |
|---|---|
| Orphan | 0.1 |
| Illness | 0.4 |
| Control | 0.0 |
| **Average** | **0.2** |

**Table 6.44  Leisure time.**

|         | Mean |
|---------|------|
| Orphan  | 4.4  |
| Illness | 3.0  |
| Control | 5.3  |
| **Average** | **4.4** |

## *Conclusion*

In Bergville, as in many South African communities, HIV will impact on an already poor society. Many children's parents already live away from home. Many children are not attending school. Measuring the economic impact of illness has been difficult, but the impact of a death of a household member is clear and large.

Illness does, however, appear to have a negative impact on the realisation of children's rights. Children living in households containing ill adults are more likely not to attend school than children from orphan or control households. This is at present mainly a result of child illness, in addition to the economic strain faced by all the households.

The care of orphaned children by their grandparents appears to lessen the impact of death on children. A higher proportion of children in orphan households attended school. Consumption, in part, was affected by high levels of expenditure on funerals, but expenditure on food and education appeared relatively stable compared to control households. Although such findings are encouraging, the sustainability is questionable. Many of the orphaned households had sold assets to mitigate the short-term financial impact. In the long term this may have serious negative implications, particularly if the assets were productive. Households also borrowed money. As the epidemic progresses, and as deaths become more common, the capacity of family and friends to lend will be eroded and interest rates of micro lenders may increase.

Adult illness and death, within a household, have a number of serious economic, psychological and social impacts on child members.

# References

Ainsworth, M., L. Fransen and M. (eds). Over. 1997. *Confronting AIDS: Public Priorities in a Global Epidemic*. World Bank Policy Research Report. Oxford: Oxford University Press.

Barnett, T. and A. Whiteside. 2002. 'Poverty and HIV/AIDS: Impact, Coping and Mitigation Policy'. Paper prepared for UNICEF Innocenti Research Centre, Florence.

Bechu, N. 1998. The Impact of AIDS on the Economy of Families in Cote d'Ivoire: Changes in Consumption Among AIDS-Affected Households. In *Confronting AIDS: Evidence from the Developing World: Selected Background Papers for the World Bank Policy Research Report*, M. Ainsworth, L. Fransen and M. Over (eds). United Kingdom: European Commission.

Cohen, D. 1998. 'Poverty and HIV/AIDS in Sub-Saharan Africa'. United Nations Development Program, HIV and Development Program. Issues Paper 27. New York.

Foster, S. 1996. 'The Socioeconomic Impact of HIV/AIDS in Monze District, Zambia'. Unpublished PhD thesis, Department of Public Health and Policy, London School of Hygiene and Tropical Medicine, October.

Kwaramba, P. 1998. 'The Socioeconomic Impact of HIV/AIDS on Communal Agricultural Systems in Zimbabwe'. Economic Advisory Project, Working Paper Number 19. Friedrich Ebert Stiftung, Belgravia.

Liwuhla, G. 1998. Variability in Savings and Assistance Behaviour in Households Across Ethnic Groups in Kagera Region, Tanzania. In *Confronting AIDS: Evidence from the Developing World: Selected Background Papers for the World Bank Policy Research Report*, M. Ainsworth, L. Fransen and M. Over (eds). United Kingdom: European Commission.

Loewenson, R. 1998. *Impact of HIV/AIDS: Zimbabwe*. Geneva: World Health Organisation.

Menon, R., M. Wawer, J. Konde-Luli, N. Sewankhambo and C. Li. 1998. 'The Economic Impact of Adult Mortality on Households in Rakai District Uganda'. In *Confronting AIDS: Evidence from the Developing World: Selected Background Papers for the World Bank Policy Research Report*, M. Ainsworth, L. Fransen and M. Over (eds). United Kingdom: European Commission.

Mutangadura, G. 2000. 'Household Welfare Impacts of Adult Females in Zimbabwe: Implications for Policy and Program Development'. Paper presented at the AIDS and Economics Symposium, International AIDS and Economics Network (IAEN) Symposium, Durban, July.

Nampanya-Serpell, N. 2000. 'Social and Economic Risk Factors for HIV/AIDS-Affected Families in Zambia'. Paper presented at the AIDS and Economics Symposium, International AIDS and Economics Network (IAEN) Symposium, Durban, July.

Rugalema, G. 1999. 'Adult Mortality as Entitlement Failure: AIDS and the Crisis of Rural Livelihoods in a Tanzanian Village'. PhD thesis, Institute of Social Studies, The Hague.

# PART TWO

# Interventions

/ PART TWO

/ INTERROGATIONS

CHAPTER 7

# Mitigating the Impacts with a Focus on Government Responses

*Judith Streak*

## Introduction

First, the government's policies and planning measures to mitigate the impact of HIV/AIDS on children is discussed. It is divided into three sections. The first section describes the most significant policy planning document that government has developed (in consultation with non-governmental structures) to guide its initiatives directed at mitigating the impact of HIV/AIDS on children. This is the National Integrated Plan for Children Infected and Affected by HIV/AIDS (IP) that was developed early in 2000. It also puts this into the context of the HIV/AIDS/STD Strategic Plan (2000–2005) (HIVSP). In describing the IP, the focus is on one of the programmes in it, the home- and community-based care and support programme. Section two details the nature of the model of home- and community-based support and care that the Department of Social Development (Welfare) is proposing as a basis for the design and implementation of models of care and support in provinces. It also places the chosen approach in the context of recent research results on the cost-effectiveness of different models. Section three discusses another significant initiative aimed at mitigating the impact of HIV/AIDS on children – the proposed programme to provide Nevirapine to HIV-positive pregnant women.

Second, expenditure and budget issues in government's response to the impact of HIV/AIDS on children are analysed. It does four things. First, it discusses what information is available, highlighting the extent and nature of the information problems undermining the attempt to get a detailed picture of what government has been spending on mitigating the impact of HIV/AIDS on children and what it is planning to spend over the Medium Term

Expenditure Framework (MTEF) period. Second, it presents the data on national government's total allocations to HIV/AIDS over the MTEF. Third, it analyses the budget allocations to the IP. Finally, it looks at the real trend in the budget allocations to social security payments over the period 2000/01–2003/04. The aim of the latter is to indicate whether government has been budgeting for the increased demand for social security payments that is implied by its approach to caring for orphans and other children made vulnerable by HIV/AIDS.

Third, the service delivery problems that are being experienced are examined. These include the implementation of the Integrated Plan/Strategy, the delay in the provision of Nevirapine to HIV-positive pregnant women and in the problems preventing orphans from accessing social security payments. Government's policy initiatives to mitigate the impact of HIV/AIDS on children and budget allocations will do nothing if the plans are not implemented quickly and effectively. It is clear that a number of service delivery challenges will have to be overcome if the plans and budget allocations are to have an impact and ensure that children's rights are protected.

The conclusion highlights urgent information needs in order to understand better, and monitor, what government is doing to mitigate the impacts of HIV/AIDS on children.

## *Government's policy response: Plans of action*
### The primary plans

Piecing together the story regarding which government policy and planning documents are driving government's response to the impact of HIV/AIDS on children is difficult. This is because there are so many initiatives that have evolved and because the approach is such that it involves input and collaboration from three leading departments – health, education and social development. Another factor is that although the policy/planning initiatives are theoretically led by national government it is difficult to know whether provinces have their own planning documents and what they are. From telephone conversations with representatives of the Department of Social Development (Welfare) and the National HIV/STD Directorate of the Department of Health and scanning the literature the following was concluded: government's mitigation attempts for children are being led by an implementation document titled the National Integrated Plan for Children Infected and Affected by HIV/AIDS (IP); and this, in turn, is guided by the broader HIV/AIDS/STD Strategic Plan for South Africa 2000–2005 (HIVSP). It is necessary to note two things. First, the initiatives in the IP are probably not the only initiatives that government is involved in to mitigate the impact of HIV/AIDS on children. Second, whilst the programmes in the IP are targeted mainly at children, children do not constitute the entire target group of the IP.

## The HIV/AIDS/STD Strategic Plan for South Africa 2000–2005 (HIVSP)

The purpose of this plan is to guide the country's response to the epidemic. It is not only a plan for the health sector, but a statement of intent for the country as a whole. It recognises that no single sector, ministry, department or organisation is solely responsible for addressing the HIV epidemic. It envisages that all government departments, organisations and stakeholders will use the HIVSP as the basis to develop their own strategic and operational plans so that all initiatives can be harmonised to maximise efficiency and effectiveness (Department of Health, 2000).

## The National Integrated Plan for Children Infected and Affected by HIV/AIDS (IP)

The overall goal of the IP is 'to ensure access to an appropriate and effective integrated system of prevention, care and support services for children infected and affected by HIV/AIDS' (Departments of Health, Social Development and Education, 2000). This goal was to be achieved through four main programmes:

Programme 1: community-based care and support;
Programme 2: strengthening voluntary counselling and testing (VCT) initiatives;
Programme 3: life skills and HIV/AIDS education in primary and secondary schools;
Programme 4: community outreach/community mobilisation.

Programme 1 involved the development of strategies for care of orphans and community-based models of care for people living with HIV/AIDS, focusing on policy development and the piloting of approaches.

Programme 4 involves community-based HIV/AIDS awareness programmes to link and promote the other three initiatives. This programme provides the thread that will link the other programmes together. It aims to focus on raising the level of awareness amongst community leaders of HIV/AIDS in general, existing and new HIV/AIDS programmes, and activities in the community on how to access services related to HIV/AIDS.

The executive summary of the IP describes the four programmes as follows: 'The programmes will include the development of co-ordinating structures, income generation activities, specific prevention activities targeting children and youth, community-based care, capacity building, access to grants and legal placements, training of teachers, as well as voluntary counselling and testing. These initiatives will be underpinned by a community outreach programme aimed at increased HIV/AIDS awareness' (Departments of Health, Education and Welfare, 2000).

As regards the relative importance of the programmes, the decision was for the life skills programme in schools to be the core of the initiative. Developing strategies for the care of orphans and community- and home-based models of care for people living with HIV would form a smaller component. Strengthening current efforts to make available VCT facilities would also form a smaller component (Departments of Education, Health and Social Development, 2000).

The explicit programme objectives of the IP/IS were:

- establishing and implementing integrated community-based care and support programmes for children infected and affected by HIV/AIDS;
- improving access to VCT services for 12.5 per cent of the population aged 15–49 over three years focussing on youth and rural communities;
- implementing the life skills and HIV/AIDS education programme in 20 per cent of primary and secondary schools in the first year, a further 40 per cent the next year, and 40 per cent in year three, ensuring 100 per cent coverage by 2002/03;
- mobilising communities through community-based HIV/AIDS awareness programmes.

Following the umbrella guidelines of the HIVSP, an inter-sectoral and inter-departmental approach was promoted for implementation of the IP. The role of the planning document is to give guidelines to provinces. Provinces are supposed to develop their own implementation plans within the principles and guidelines stipulated in the national plan (Departments of Education, Health and Welfare, 2000). The departments that are to take the lead in implementation are Health, Social Development (Welfare) and Education.

It is acknowledged that successful implementation of the plan requires a great deal of communication and co-ordination between the different spheres of government, the different departments at the provincial level and between families, communities and government. This is particularly the case in the home- and community-based care and support programme. It involves Health and Social Development (Welfare) departments in provinces taking lead roles in projects. It involves families and community structures being involved in providing medical and other forms of care.

The planning document envisages implementation over a three-year period, beginning in 2000/01. But, all of the programmes were not on the agenda for all of the provinces in year one. In 2000/01, the strategy was to be implemented in its entirety (all four programmes) in three provinces, namely Eastern Cape, Mpumalanga and Northern Province. North West, Free State and Northern Cape were to implement three of the four programmes (namely life skills, VCT, and community-based care and support). Gauteng, Western Cape and KwaZulu-Natal were to implement the life skills and VCT programmes only (Departments of Education, Health and Welfare, 2000). A district approach is being followed meaning that only one district per province was to see implementation of the plan (or the components thereof that it had decided would be implemented in that province). To summarise: the initial plan was to implement the whole strategy (all four programmes) in one district in three provinces, three of the four programmes in the strategy in one district in six provinces and two programmes in one district in three provinces. The aim in the initial planning document was to extend all four programmes in every province in districts of need over year two and three of the strategy. By the end of the three year period, it was envisaged that provinces would take financial responsibility for the programmes in the IP (developing them further according to need) while districts would take the lead role in delivery.

**Three changes made to the initial plan since its inception**
First, an extra year has been added to the initial three-year trial and national government financed period. Now, national government is to finance the project until the end of 2003/04. (Department of Treasury, 2001a).

Second, two of the programmes in the IP/IS have been merged: the community-based care and support programme and the community outreach programme. The title of this programme is now the home- and community-based care and support programme (HCBCS). The decision to integrate the two programmes flowed from early experience in the pilots in the six districts trying to implement the plan and the obvious conceptual flaw in leaving out the programme designed to link the other three programmes in the strategy in three of the initial pilot districts. In the end, the first year of the plan saw the initial implementation of the entire strategy, encompassing the life skills programme, voluntary counselling and testing, and home- and community-based care and support, in six pilot sites. The pilot sites were in Mpumalanga, Eastern Cape, North West, Northern Province, Free State and Northern Cape. Western Cape, KwaZulu-Natal and Gauteng were only involved in the VCT and life skills programmes.

Third, there have been changes to the models that the plan suggests implementing institutions draw on, in conceptualising their chosen models of care. The initial plan did not advocate the use of any one model. It simply mentions that effective models of care and support must:

- take into account the need to address the immediate issues of poverty as they relate to basic needs and resources; and to facilitate and enable sustainable development and income generation which can address medium- and longer-term issues of poverty;
- address the needs of the most vulnerable people, for example, older persons, children, women and people with disabilities;
- support and facilitate the delivery of services and build the capacity of communities, especially non-governmental and community-based organisations.

## Government expenditures to mitigate the impact of HIV/AIDS on children
### Difficulties in estimation

The search for information on what government has been, and is planning to spend, on mitigating the impact of HIV/AIDS on children ended with some success but a lot of disappointment.

The IP is being financed by the national revenue fund via a special allocation called the Integrated Strategy (IS) allocation. The money is shared between the Health, Welfare and Education sectors and appears on the budgets of the national Departments of Health, Social Development and Education. It is in turn allocated to the provincial Departments of Health, Social Development and Education in the nine provinces for spending on each of the three programmes. The funds are flowing to provinces in the form of three conditional grants for each province. Because conditional grants are recorded in the National Budget Review, the National Estimates of Expenditure, and each province's Provincial Estimates of Expenditure, it is possible to estimate how much is being allocated to the programmes in the IP. Aside from the fact that these three documents do not provide information on the allocations for the outer two years in the MTEF cycle, it is possible to detail budget allocations falling under the banner of the IP/IS. But, the IS fund is not the only mechanism through which government money is being spent. It proved impossible to get adequate information on how much government money flows through other channels. The other channels, for which data is currently not available, are listed below.

EXPLICIT ALLOCATIONS TO THE IP AND OTHER HIV/AIDS
PROGRAMMES BY PROVINCIAL GOVERNMENTS
Provinces are explicitly allocating money for programmes directed at preventing and mitigating the HIV/AIDS epidemic over and above that which is being spent by them from the national government special IS allocation. This

may be for spending on the programmes in the IP or on different programmes. Whilst data on how much a couple of provinces allocated this year to HIV/AIDS programmes was available, the data is sketchy. Moreover, no province was able to provide data for child-specific HIV/AIDS programmes or for spending plans beyond this financial year. The national Department of Treasury is planning a study on the fiscal impacts of HIV/AIDS. As part of this process, provincial Health, Social Development and Education departments have been requested to collate and provide it with information on what their departments are planning to spend – explicitly –on prevention and mitigation efforts. Perhaps once this process is complete, it will be easier to piece together a picture of what provinces are spending on HIV/AIDS and on mitigating the impact of HIV/AIDS on children.

IMPLICIT ALLOCATIONS BY NATIONAL AND PROVINCIAL GOVERNMENTS

Funds are being implicitly spent by government due to increased demand placed by HIV/AIDS impacts on public services. For example, resources are being diverted to patients with HIV/AIDS-related illnesses in paediatric wards. In the words of the Department of Treasury: 'The HIV/AIDS epidemic represents a major threat . . . Public finances will be impacted through the increased need for medical services, expanding provincial health expenditure and the increased cost of delivering social services as a result of the loss of qualified staff' (Department of Treasury, 2001a). There are no data estimates on what departments such as health and education spend implicitly on mitigating the impact of HIV/AIDS on all users and on children in particular.

IMPLICIT AND EXPLICIT ALLOCATIONS VIA SOCIAL GRANTS AND POVERTY RELIEF FUNDS

Aside from providing free education and healthcare, government's other responsibility is income support. This can be further broken down into two categories: provision of grants to orphans and their caregivers; and provision of start-up finance for income-generating projects.

Theoretically therefore, information is needed on how much money has been flowing to children made vulnerable by HIV/AIDS and their caregivers through the social security budgets of provinces, and through the national government's poverty relief fund. This information is not provided in the budget documents and could not be obtained through conversations with representatives of government. Moreover, this information was requested from the national Departments of Social Development and Treasury but both were unable to provide it.

IMPLICIT AND EXPLICIT ALLOCATIONS VIA ALLOCATIONS TO GOVERNMENT AND NGO-RUN RESIDENTIAL CARE FACILITIES FOR CHILDREN

Data is needed not only on how much has been going to care facilities run by the government, but also by non-governmental organisations (NGOs). Again, budgets are not constructed in a way that allows this information to be extrapolated and the national Departments of Treasury and Social Development were not able to provide this information.

GOVERNMENT EXPENDITURE ON THE PROGRAMME TO REDUCE VERTICAL TRANSMISSION FROM MOTHER TO CHILD

Government is spending money supplemented by donor funding. The budget documents do not, however, provide any indication of how much is allocated for this programme. Hence, data was collected from provincial Departments of Health, and only one, the Western Cape Department of Health, has allocated money. This totalled R6.1 million in 2001/02.

**Summary**

The difficulty in gathering information on budgeting for HIV/AIDS is surprising in light of the fact that structures have been set up – under the direction of the HIVSP – that imply ease in accessing this information.

The Interdepartmental Committee on AIDS (IDC) consists of representatives from all government departments who co-ordinate HIV/AIDS activities. The IDC meets monthly. Goals of the IDC include facilitating the development of HIV/AIDS workplace policies ensuring that all departments allocate financial resources to HIV/AIDS and develop minimum HIV/AIDS programmes (Department of Health, 2000a and 2000b).

One of the goals of the IDC, that was established to monitor the country's progress in responding to the epidemic, is to ensure that all government departments allocated sufficient resources to HIV/AIDS. This implies collection, analysis and dissemination of data. Two other structures that have been set up to co-ordinate and monitor the implementation of government, community and family initiatives also suggest ease in collecting the types of funding flows outlined above. These are the National Directorate on HIV/AIDS and the provincial co-ordinating committees.

**Approach to estimation**

On the basis of the information constraints outlined above, the approach taken in describing how much has been and is being set aside by government for spending on mitigating the impact of HIV/AIDS on children is as follows:

*Mitigating the Impacts* . . . 155

1. how much national government has allocated for spending on HIV/AIDS is presented;
2. budget allocations to the IS/IP are examined;
3. sketchy and unclear data collected informally on how much additional money has been set aside by provinces for spending on HIV/AIDS in 2001 is presented;
4. trends in real terms in the social security budgets of the provinces as an indicator of the extent to which provinces (who are responsible for making social security payments) are budgeting for the impact of HIV/AIDS on welfare payments is presented.

Because the main programmes that government has put in place to mitigate the impact of HIV/AIDS are those that fall under the label IS/IP, the analysis focuses on the IS allocations, giving some idea of how much is being spent on mitigating impacts on children. However, in focusing on the IS funding it must be remembered that other money is being allocated through the five channels outlined above. It must also be remembered that some of the money spent on the IS will not flow to children (for example, VCT is for the target population 15–49 years of age).

**National budget allocations to HIV/AIDS**
The Budget documents provide estimates of the total allocation to HIV/AIDS at the national level. It works out to be a small portion of the total national health budget, which was R6.611 billion for 2001/02 (Department of Treasury, 2001a and 2000b).

**The official conservative estimate**
The conservative estimate, which is presented in a statement in the Budget Review is R236 million for 2001/02, increasing to R416 million in 2002/03 and R423.5 million in 2003/04. This is comprised of the special allocation to the IS and the allocation (through the Department of Health), to Government's Aids Action Programme. This conservative estimate of national government expenditure on HIV/AIDS is 3.5 per cent of the total national health expenditure for 2001/02. Table 7.1 presents the conservative budget allocations (real and nominal) to HIV/AIDS from national government for the MTEF period.

**Table 7.1 National budget allocations to HIV/AIDS, 2001/02–2003/04 (R millions).**

|  | 2001/02 | 2002/03 | 2003/04 |
|---|---|---|---|
| Integrated Strategy (special allocation) | R125.0 | R300.0 | R304.5 |
| Government Aids Action Plan (on budget of National Department of Health) | R111.4 | R116.0 | R119.0 |
| Total budget allocation to HIV/AIDS | R236.4 | R416.0 | R423.5 |
| Real value – 2000 rands | R223.4 | R375.8 | R366.2 |

Source: Department of Treasury, (2001a and 2001b)
Note: The Department of Treasury's estimates of CPI inflation, presented in the 2001 Budget Review are used to deflate with 2000/01 as the base year.

**A larger more inclusive estimate**

A more inclusive estimate is reached when one examines the money that flows from the three relevant departments (Health, Social Development and Education) in the Estimates of National Expenditure and includes TB expenditure as part of expenditure on HIV/AIDS. The total national allocation is made up of two sources of funding:

- the special allocation to the IS strategy, of which the total amount is allocated to, and appears on, the budgets of the national Departments of Health, Social Development and Education;
- allocations on national department's regular budgets in addition to the IS money.

This implies that to get an estimate of the amount being allocated at national level to HIV/AIDS it is necessary to look at the estimated budgets of each of the three departments that are given in the Estimates of National Expenditure 2001.

With this approach we reach the conclusion that close to R300 million is allocated for 2001/02 (R295.8 exactly), comprised of the flows of funding as outlined in Figure 7.1. This estimate is 4.46 per cent of the total national health budget for 2001/02.

**Budget allocations to the IP**

As is illustrated in Figure 7.1 a large portion (42 per cent) of the total moneys that national Government has allocated to HIV/AIDS in 2001/02 is allocated to the IS Fund for the implementation of the IP. Table 7.2 shows the nominal allocations to the IS fund and real allocations based on the Department of

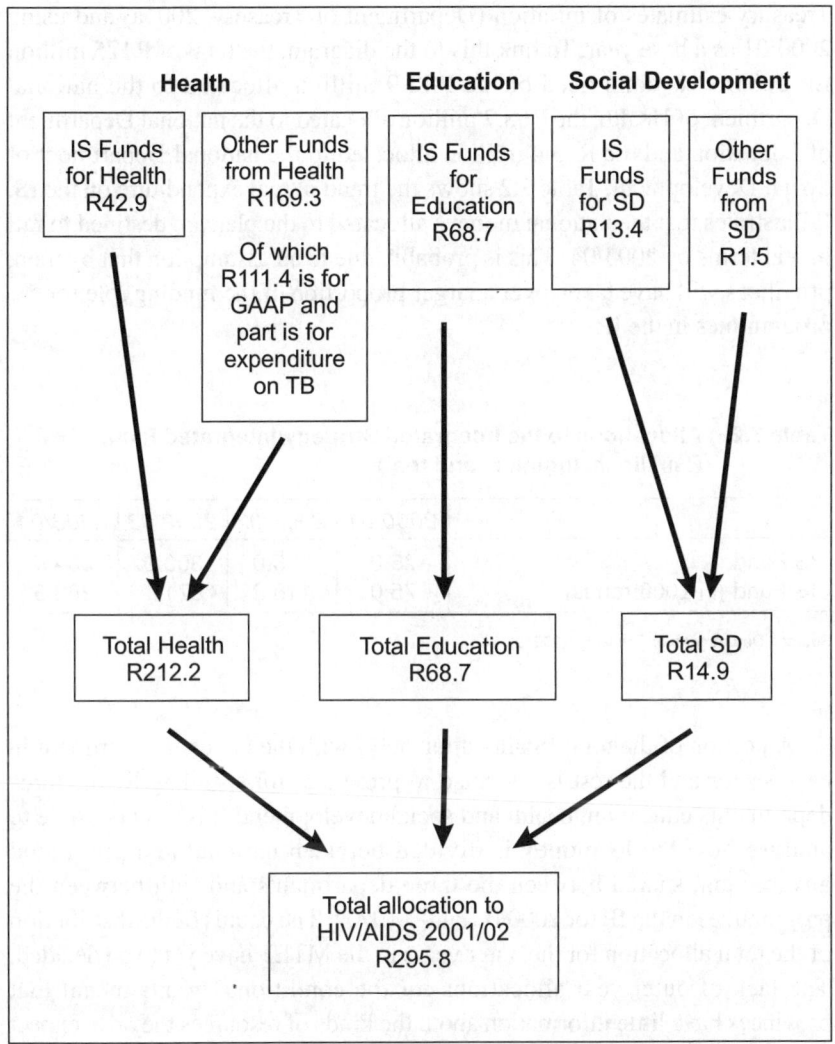

Figure 7.1 Inclusive estimate of national allocation to HIV/AIDS in 2001/02 (R million).

Treasury estimates of inflation (Department of Treasury, 2001a) and using 2000/01 as a base year. To link this to the diagram, the total of R125 million for 2001/02 is comprised of the R42.9 million allocated to the national Department of Health, the R68.7 million allocated to the national Department of Education and the R13.4 million allocated to the national Department of Social Development. Table 7.2 shows the trend in real expenditure on the IS. It illustrates that the national moneys allocated to the plan are destined to fall in real terms by 2003/04. This is probably due to an assumption that by then, provinces will have taken over a larger proportion of the funding role for the programmes in the IP.

**Table 7.2 Allocations to the Integrated Strategy/Integrated Plan, R millions, (nominal and real).**

|  | 2000/01 | 2001/02 | 2002/03 | 2003/04 |
|---|---|---|---|---|
| IS Fund | 75.0 | 125.0 | 300.0 | 304.5 |
| IS Fund (in 2000 rands) | 75.0 | 118.3 | 271.1 | 263.3 |

Source: Department of Treasury (2001a)

A portion of the total IS allocation stays with the national department in each sector and the rest is allocated to provinces for spending by the three departments education, health and social development. It is only possible to analyse how the IS money is divided between national and provincial government, shared between the three departments and split between the programmes in the IP for 2000/01 and 2001/02. The details of the distribution of the total allocation for the outer years in the MTEF have yet to be decided. The lack of outer year allocations for the conditional grants meant that provinces have little information about the kinds of resources they can expect to receive in future years of the programme(s) (Hickey and Whelan, 2001).

In 2000 65 per cent of the IS allocation money was given to provinces (via conditional grants). In 2001 there was an increase in the role of provinces. Their share increased to 88 per cent. Provinces received R110 million of the R125 million. The increased devolution of responsibility may be a cause for concern as provinces continue to be unable to spend a number of other application-based conditional grants and struggled to spend the money given to them for the IP last year. It is unknown how much of 2000 IS funds transferred to provinces went unspent. According to representatives of the national Department of Social Development's HIV Unit and the HIV/AIDS Directorate in the national Department of Health, the six national Departments of Health and Social Development had problems with spending their allocations in 2000/01. Only at the end of the financial year had all the funds given to the provincial Departments of Social Development been allocated to delivery institutions. The Chief Directorate of HIV/AIDS and STDs in the national Department of Health has also relayed that the provincial Departments of Health had problems spending the R16.8 million that was allocated to them. The nature of the problems causing this under spending is discussed below. Of the R110.1 million allocated to provinces in 2001/02, R63.5 million is allocated to the provincial Departments of Education. R34.1 million is allocated to Departments of Health and R12 million to Departments of Social Development (Department of Treasury, 2001).

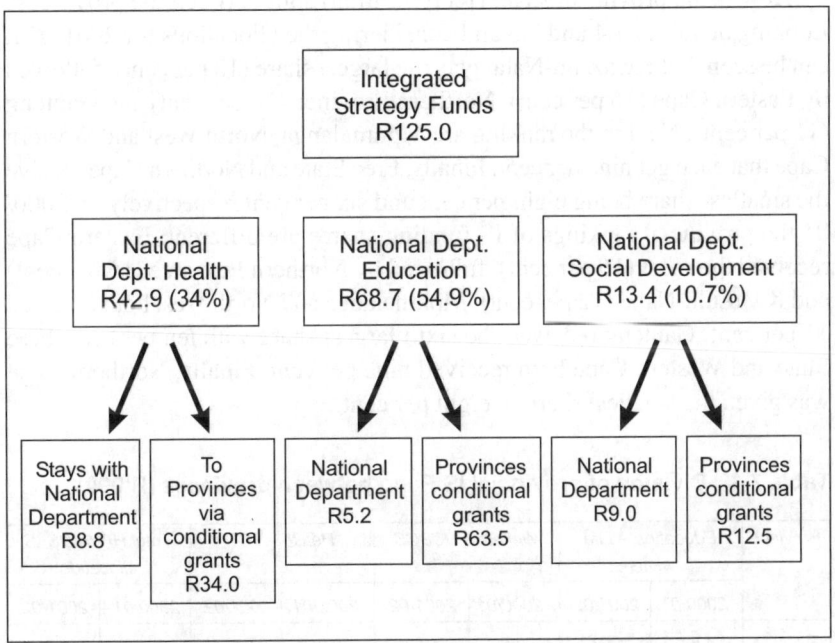

Figure 7.2 How the IS money is shared between national and provincial governments and sectors for 2001/02 (R millions).

Table 7.3 outlines the programme distribution of the IS money. It shows that most of the money is allocated to the life skills programme. The remainder is split almost equally between the other two programmes: voluntary counselling and testing, and home- and community-based care scheme.

**Table 7.3 Allocation of Integrated Strategy Fund by programme (R'000 & %).**

|  | 2000/01 | 2001/02 | 2001/02 in 2000 Rands | Share of total in 2000/01 | Share of total in 2001/02 | Real growth 2000/01–2001/02 |
|---|---|---|---|---|---|---|
| Life skills | 39 000 | 71 000 | 67 235 | 52% | 57% | 72% |
| VCT | 20 200 | 26 000 | 24 621 | 27% | 21% | 22% |
| HCBCS | 15 700 | 28 000 | 26 515 | 21% | 22% | 69% |
| Total | 74 900 | 125 000 | 118 371 | 100% | 100% | 58% |

Source: Hickey and Whelan (2001)

How is the provincial share (R110 million) split between the provinces? Looking at Tables 7.4 and 7.5 and considering the allocations for 2001/02 it can be seen that KwaZulu-Natal gets the largest share (18 per cent), followed by Eastern Cape (16 per cent), Northern Province (14 per cent) and Gauteng (11 per cent). Next in the ranking are Mpumalanga, North West and Western Cape that each get nine per cent. Finally, Free State and Northern Cape receive the smallest share being eight per cent and six per cent respectively. In 2000/01 the provincial rankings of IS funding shares are different: Eastern Cape received the most (16 per cent), followed by Northern Province (15 per cent) and KwaZulu-Natal (12 per cent). Mpumalanga and North West both received 11 per cent. Gauteng received the sixth largest share with ten per cent. Free State and Western Cape both received nine per cent. Finally, Northern Cape was given the smallest share of eight per cent.

**Table 7.4 Division of provincial IS Fund between provinces (R'000).**

| Province | Education – Life skills | | Welfare – HCBCS | | Health – VCT | | Total HIV/AIDS IS allocation | |
|---|---|---|---|---|---|---|---|---|
|  | 2000/01 | 2001/02 | 2000/01 | 2001/02 | 2000/01 | 2001/02 | 2000/01 | 2001/02 |
| EC | 4 572 | 11 747 | 950 | 1 500 | 2 213 | 3 850 | 7 735 | 17 097 |
| FS | 2 297 | 4 001 | 910 | 1 500 | 1 460 | 3 850 | 4 667 | 9 351 |
| G | 2 296 | 7 810 |  | 1 000 | 2 486 | 3 500 | 4 782 | 12 310 |
| KZN | 4 617 | 14 033 |  | 1 500 | 1 500 | 4 500 | 6 117 | 20 033 |
| M | 2 473 | 4 636 | 960 | 1 500 | 1 822 | 3 350 | 5 255 | 9 486 |
| NC | 1 467 | 1 207 | 1 000 | 1 500 | 1 239 | 3 850 | 3 706 | 6 557 |
| NP | 4 572 | 9 969 | 800 | 1 500 | 1 903 | 3 850 | 7 275 | 15 319 |
| NW | 2 339 | 5 080 | 1 000 | 1 500 | 2 006 | 3 850 | 5 345 | 10 430 |
| WC | 2 297 | 5 017 |  | 1 000 | 2 190 | 3 500 | 4 487 | 9 517 |
| Total | 26 930 | 63 500 | 5 620 | 12 500 | 16 819 | 34 100 | 49 369 | 110 100 |

Source: Department of Treasury (2001a)

**Table 7.5  Division of provincial IS Funds between provinces (%).**

| Province | Education – Life skills | | Welfare – HCBCS | | Health – VCT and HCBS | | Total HIV/AIDS IS allocation | |
|---|---|---|---|---|---|---|---|---|
| | 2000/01 | 2001/02 | 2000/01 | 2001/02 | 2000/01 | 2001/02 | 2000/01 | 2001/02 |
| EC | 17 | 18 | 17 | 12 | 13 | 11 | 16 | 16 |
| FS | 9 | 6 | 16 | 12 | 9 | 11 | 9 | 8 |
| G | 9 | 12 | 0 | 8 | 15 | 10 | 10 | 11 |
| KZN | 17 | 22 | 0 | 12 | 9 | 13 | 12 | 18 |
| M | 9 | 7 | 17 | 12 | 11 | 10 | 11 | 9 |
| NC | 5 | 2 | 18 | 12 | 7 | 11 | 8 | 6 |
| NP | 17 | 16 | 14 | 12 | 11 | 11 | 15 | 14 |
| NW | 9 | 8 | 18 | 12 | 12 | 11 | 11 | 9 |
| WC | 9 | 8 | 0 | 8 | 13 | 10 | 9 | 9 |

Source: Department of Treasury (2001a)

What criteria were used to distribute the provincial share of the IS funds between provinces? Different criteria were used for each of the three conditional grants. The provincial shares of IS funding presented above were thus a product of three formula/criteria applied by the three national departments: Social Development, Health and Education.

Looking first at Social Development, Table 7.4 shows that in 2000/01 the six provinces that received money for the HCBCS pilots received almost the same allocation. Furthermore, in 2001/02, the amounts allocated are exactly the same, except for the case of Gauteng and Western Cape, that receive R0.5 million less than the other seven provinces. According to a representative of the national Social Development's HIV Directorate heavily involved in assisting provinces with implementation of the HCBCS leg of the IP, the reason Western Cape, Gauteng and KwaZulu-Natal did not receive funding in 2000/01 is because they already had many support and care initiatives. It appears as if in 2001/02 the lack of current initiatives was also the main criteria for the distribution of IS funds.

It is important to point out that because provincial Departments of Health and Social Development are jointly responsible for the piloting of the HCBCS part of the IS, some of the money allocated to provincial health departments for the IP will be spent on HCBCS and hence flow to orphans. What criteria have been used for the provincial distribution of the health component of the provincial IS funds? According to the Department of Treasury (2001a) the distribution was based on the national survey conducted in 1999 on the status and availability of VCT in all provinces and the business plans submitted by the provinces. Other reliable information sources tell a different story. According to these, the national Department of Health took provincial capacity into account in their formula, and also considered the urgency of the epidemic – as measured by HIV prevalence rates.

The education component of the IS provincial funds was simply allocated between provinces by copying the formula used to calculate the education component of the provincial equitable share.

The IS/IP was launched in 2000/01. National government has budgeted for the strategy for four years, but thereafter, 'Provinces will need to make provision to sustain all activities and initiatives . . . as part of their line function budgets' (Departments of Education, Health and Social Development, 2000).

**The little known about provinces budgeting for HIV/AIDS projects**

The national allocations to mitigating the impact of HIV/AIDS are being supplemented by substantial additional flows of funds from provincial budgets. The total provincial allocations to HIV/AIDS in 20001/02 was R111.1 million. The sketchy picture that can be drawn from these flows of money for 2001/02 is shown in Table 7.6.

Table 7.6  Provincial HIV/AIDS allocation for 2001/02 and department (if known).

| | | | |
|---|---|---|---|
| Gauteng | R72 million | All departments | |
| Western Cape | R23.6 million | Health | |
| Northern Province | R2 million | Health | |
| Mpumalanga | R3 million | Health | |
| Free State | R3 million | Health | |
| Eastern Cape | ? | | |
| KwaZulu-Natal | R7.5 million | Health R4 m | Welfare R3.5 m |
| Northern Cape | ? | | |
| North West | ? | | |

Source: Personal conversations with provincial co-ordinators of the HIV/AIDS programme in the departments of health or other representatives from provincial departments of health

**The impact of HIV/AIDS in provincial welfare budgets**

The key tasks in child care and support programmes are accessing welfare benefits, maintaining children in school, and ensuring that basic necessities such as food and clothes are provided (Russell and Schneider, 2000).

Providing social security payments to children and their caregivers forms a part of the strategy in government's chosen approach to mitigating the impact of HIV/AIDS on children. The home- and community-based approaches which are being used to protect orphans implies that the government will not only be responsible for delivering key social services to them, but also for providing income support through the social security budget and poverty alleviation projects in communities affected by HIV/AIDS.

It was not possible to get information on how much has been spent on the three child-specific grants and how much has been budgeted for them over the MTEF period. There is no alternative but to look at all social security expenditure as an indicator of the extent to which provinces are budgeting for HIV/AIDS impacts. This means that these indicators include expenditure on grants other than those specifically targeted at children.

Table 7.7 Provincial social security budgets, 2000/01 and MTEF period (R'000).

|  | 2000/01 | 2001/02 | 2002/03 | 2003/04 |
|---|---|---|---|---|
| EC | 3 853 537 | 4 322 315 | 4 244 627 | 4 588 724 |
| FS | 1 119 566 | 1 202 751 | 1 309 068 | 1 405 849 |
| G | 2 176 907 | 2 306 431 | 2 470 766 | 2 619 005 |
| KZN | 4 142 243 | 4 248 096 | 4 837 138 | 5 365 030 |
| M | 1 117 468 | 1 448 029 | 1 614 576 | 1 666 264 |
| NC | 589 085 | 582 666 | 609 718 | 633 567 |
| NP | 2 440 354 | 2 605 052 | 2 848 873 | 3 179 555 |
| NW | 1 601 684 | 1 798 820 | 2 044 016 | 2 155 831 |
| WC | 1 862 950 | 1 919 132 | 2 076 602 | 2 236 791 |
| Total | 18 903 794 | 20 433 292 | 22 055 384 | 23 850 616 |

Source: Provincial estimates of expenditure (2001/02–2003/04) and J. Adams (2001)

Table 7.8 Real growth rates in social security budgets, 2000/01–2003/04, (%).

| EC | 2.9% |
|---|---|
| FS | 8.5% |
| G | 4.0% |
| KZN | 11.4% |
| M | 28.9% |
| NC | −7.0% |
| NP | 12.6% |
| NW | 16.3% |
| WC | 3.8% |

Source: Provincial estimates of expenditure (2001/02–2003/04), J. Adams (2001) and Department of Treasury (2001a) for CPI inflation projections and calculations

It can be seen that all provinces, except Northern Cape, have budgets for social security payments over the next three years that increase in real terms compared to 2000/01. However, this does not imply that they will be able to absorb the increased demand for social security by children implied by HIV/AIDS impacts (on the assumption that service delivery is improved). The overwhelming majority of the social security budget is spent on non-children-specific grants – the pension (old age grant) and disability grant. In 2000/01, pension payments constituted 67 per cent of total provincial expenditure on grants, disability payments 23 per cent, child support grant payments five per cent, foster grant payments two per cent, care dependency payments one per cent and maintenance payments one per cent (the maintenance grant has now been phased out). In other words, the old age and disability grants comprise just over 90 per cent of total social security expenditure and child-specific grants just under ten per cent. The outer two years of the MTEF will also see inflation-linked increases to the five primary grants. At the same time, the impact of HIV/AIDS on poor households will ensure that the number of people that want to access the two grants that take such a large chunk of the social security budget will increase. It is these factors that make it seem unlikely that the provinces have budgeted sufficiently for the increased need to make social security payments to orphans.

## *Difficulties and problems in government's attempts to alleviate the impact of HIV/AIDS on children*
### Problems in implementing the IP/IS
'The strong emphasis on the need for an integrated plan has been noted. To achieve this aim is not easy as Government is structured in a way that does not foster integration' (Departments of Health, Education and Social Development, 2000).

Whilst progress in the implementation of the IP is now being made, the IP got off to a slow start in the first year of implementation (2000). All three departments responsible for implementing the IP in the provinces have been experiencing delivery problems. According to the national Department of Health's HIV/STD Directorate the following problems explain why provincial departments of health had only spent 9.3 per cent of the health conditional grant allocated to them for the implementation of the IP by March 2001 (Simelelo, 2001):

- the late publication of the IS funds in the government gazette;
- the lengthy time involved in developing the integrated business plans needed before funds can be allocated to service providers;

- lack of human resource capacity at provincial level;
- long time frames of procurement processes, especially tendering.

A couple of additional problems have caused slow implementation of the IP and they need to be overcome to fast track the delivery of the HCBCS programme in the IP. These include:

- lack of capacity and information in rural communities;
- the need for training to build capacity;
- turnover of staff;
- difficulties in accessing money from Treasury by provincial Departments of Health and Social Development in two of the six provinces that were supposed to implement all of the programmes in the IP last year.

**The delay in the implementation of the programme providing Nevirapine to HIV-positive pregnant mothers**

The Nevirapine programme involving public provision of the anti-retroviral to HIV-positive pregnant women to reduce VTMC has been in the pipeline since July 2000 when the Health Minister and provincial Members of the Executive Council approved it. Implementation of the programme was supposed to begin in 18 sites on 1 April 2001. However, just before implementation, provinces were told to put the programme on hold until Cabinet had approved the project and the Medicines Control Council had registered Nevirapine (Cullinan, 2001). On 18 April 2001 the Medicines Control Council registered the drug, removing this obstacle to implementation. Cabinet had yet to remove the other obstacle (Cullinan, 2001).

**The capacity of the community to absorb orphans**

Government has reached the conclusion that community- and family-based approaches to care for orphans, with government support, is the only viable option. Loening-Voysey and Wilson (2001) warn that it is imperative to have alternative substitute care options. This is because extended family members are often not willing or available to care, and then it is not in the best interest of the child to remain within the extended family and communities may not yet be ready to accept children orphaned by HIV/AIDS.

Stigma and discrimination of people living with AIDS poses one of the greatest threats to the successful scaling-up of community-based responses. HIV-positive mothers who are rejected and unsupported, abandon their HIV-positive babies. For many of these abandoned children, statutory residential care settings are the only option. At the root of stigma and discrimination lies fear and ignorance about HIV/AIDS (Loening-Voysey and Wilson, 2001).

Government needs to bear in mind the need for balance in its scaling up of community- and family-based models of care and support for children infected and affected by HIV/AIDS and scaling down of residential care facilities. This issue is examined more closely in the section on service delivery problems below and looks at why children are falling through the safety net during the transition phase of the switch from residential and community-based services.

**Why the social security system must be redesigned if it is to benefit orphans**

There is no information available on the extent to which the three available grants are currently serving children made vulnerable by the HIV/AIDS epidemic or on how much provinces are spending, and plan to spend, on providing these grants to orphans. What is known though is that due to general service delivery problems and shortcomings on the part of the system focused on children, the social security system is failing to reach most children, especially orphans. The inability of grants to reach many children is indicated by the national Department of Social Development data on the number of beneficiaries.

Table 7.9 Number of beneficiaries of child specific grants.

|  | Number of beneficiaries | |
|---|---|---|
|  | March 2000 | March 2001 |
| Foster grant (FG) | 49 088 | 52 642 |
| Care dependency grant (CDG) | 23 705 | 31 452 |
| Child support grant (CSG) | 201 968 | 757 728 |

Source: Department of Social Development, SOCPEN database (April 2001)

In the light of the fact that there are about four million income-poor children under the age of six and large numbers of orphans, the number of beneficiaries is still small relative to need. The nature of the service delivery problems causing these low take-up figures and preventing the support network from reaching children infected and affected by HIV/AIDS, are discussed below.

A process is currently underway to redesign the social security system, including the child specific part of it. As part of this process, in 2000, Cabinet appointed a Committee of Inquiry into a Comprehensive Social Security System to develop a framework and policy options for social security in its broad sense of social protection. The Committee was expected to present its report to Cabinet in late 2001. The committee's brief included making recommendations for the redesign of the child-specific portion of the system with particular reference to ensuring that it catches orphans. The committee has consulted with civil society in developing its recommendations. There has been talk of merging the three child-specific grants into a grant of R250 per child per month that applies to all children and having additional grants to service children with special needs such as children with particular disabilities including HIV infection and AIDS. The importance of linking income payments to free schooling and healthcare, and food vouchers has also arisen.

Around 800 000 children receive the primary CSG, although there are around 4 million children living below the poverty line. This means that only 20 per cent of children that are desperately in need of income support, receive the grant that they are entitled to. Bearing in mind the link between HIV and poverty, a large portion of the children in need and who are not receiving the grant will be suffering from the impacts of the epidemic.

Clearly, government has been making progress in trying to ensure that the grant is paid to children in need – the number of beneficiaries of the CSG increased by 275 per cent between March 2000 and March 2001. But, it is struggling in this regard. There are a number of key implementation problems explaining why so few children qualifying for the CSG are receiving it (Cassiem, et al., 2000; Thorn, 2001). They are:

- lack of transport and money to get to the relevant government social development office and start the application process (particularly in rural areas);
- lack of physical infrastructure;
- denial of the CSG because the surname of the child on the Road to Health Card is not the same as the caregiver's (a situation that is common when the primary caregiver is the grandmother);
- lack of birth certificates and identification documents;
- lack of information about the availability of the grant.

The average time taken for processing grant applications will have to be speeded up – HIV-infected children do not have the time to wait for their entitlements to improve their quality of life, and the plight of orphans is so harsh and immediate that immediate income support is crucial. In addition, the nature of the safety net has to be redesigned if government is to stay true to its plan to deliver income support to orphans. In the words of Guthri, a researcher at the Child Health Policy Unit and spokesperson for the recently established Alliance for Children's Entitlement to Social Security (ACESS): 'the current social security system is fragmented and non-comprehensive, too many children fall between the gaps' (Thorn, 2001).

The key shortcomings in the design of the social security system that are ensuring that it is unable to catch sufficient orphans are:

- The age limit on the child support grant. Only children aged six or under receive the grant but many of the orphans and other children in need are older than six.
- The need for the caregiver to supply the birth certificate of the child when applying for all the child-specific grants. After the death of a parent or parents it may be difficult to access the document.
- The nature of the process involved in deciding which children are eligible for the CDG. To become eligible for the CDG, a child has to be classified as requiring permanent home care due to his or her severe mental or physical disability. The permanent home care criteria is very exclusionary and, in practice, the decision for giving a child eligibility is subjective.
- The requirement that the FG only be given to foster caregivers after the court has placed the child in the care of these caregivers and the fact that the number of foster children is limited to six. As an example of how orphans are falling through the cracks of the social security system, the case study tells of a foster mother who is finding it difficult to access the FG for the fourteen children she is caring for.

**Designing a comprehensive social security system for all children**
In response to the many shortcomings identified in existing social security provisions, three major policy development processes have been initiated. The first of these is the Inter-Ministerial Committee of Inquiry into a comprehensive social security system. The Committee was established to consult with stakeholders and make recommendations for an improved system. In the interim, the Department of Social Development has undertaken to make amendments to the Social Assistance Act that governs the existing grants. The third process is a broad and comprehensive review of all child-related law which is being undertaken by the South African Law Commission with the aim of drafting a new Child Care Act to replace the existing Child Care Act (No. 74 of 1983).

While it would be impossible and unethical to have social assistance provisions targeted at children infected or affected by HIV/AIDS, the proposed amendments to the current social security system for children take cognisance of the fact that there is a need to ensure that these recommendations meet the needs of all vulnerable children, including those affected by the AIDS epidemic.

Two major options for an improved social security system for children have been proposed and are supported by the children's sector (National workshop on social security for children in South Africa, 2001).

The first is to increase the age limit of the child support grant from seven to 18 years and the value of the grant to a more realistic figure. Given the fact that the money is generally used to benefit the entire household, and not just the eligible child, the value of the grant to the child is diluted. Despite this, the extension of the CSG would greatly improve the situation of children.

The second major option is to introduce a basic income grant for everyone. The basic income grant would mean that every individual would have some income and, as a result, a large proportion of the poor population would move nearer to or across the poverty line.

**Alternative forms of social assistance**
Social security provisioning is currently almost entirely the burden of the Department of Social Development, with very little contribution from the other government departments. It is necessary to explore alternative forms of social assistance such as free healthcare (for all children), food vouchers, subsidised transport and free education. Those departments that do provide some form of assistance need to review the criteria governing accessibility so as to ensure that children infected/affected by AIDS can benefit. An example is the housing subsidy, which is only available to adults over the age of 21 years. Children living in child-headed households are therefore unable to access the subsidy.

**Inter-sectoral collaboration**
Poor inter-sectoral collaboration between health, welfare and home affairs has a direct impact on the administration of all grants. Corrupt officials in the Department of Home Affairs have been known to charge applicants elevated fees before issuing birth certificates, essential if the caregiver wishes to apply for a grant. Mobile home affairs offices have been cut back, and dates and times of visits are changed without prior notice to recipients (Child Health Policy Institute and Black Sash, 2000). This adds yet another stumbling block for caregivers in desperate need of social assistance.

One of the recommendations that have been made is that birth registration procedures are introduced at health facilities so as to ensure that newborns are issued with birth certificates. Caregivers would then be able to access a grant should they need one. This would require extensive collaboration between the Departments of Health and Home Affairs.

**Administrative issues**
Means testing and administration of grants require major changes so as to minimise incidence of corruption and increase the uptake of the grants. Families affected by HIV/AIDS where one or more breadwinner has died should be able to access interim financial assistance during the three or more months that it takes for the grant to be processed.

Furthermore, when a caregiver dies of AIDS, the grant is automatically cancelled. In order to avoid this, the grant should follow the child and not be registered in the name of the caregiver. Linked to this is the need to improve accessibility of the child support grant to child-headed households.

**Costs and implications for social development services**

The question remains whether any of these recommendations will be accepted and, if so, where the money will come from to finance their implementation.

The cost of extending the CSG to children up to the age of 17 years would be approximately R16.8 billion per annum. This costing was based on the assumption that the current means test is maintained, with 14 million children benefiting (Haarmann, 2001). Put in perspective, this amounts to over half of the total welfare budget for 2001/02. The cost to the Government of providing a basic income grant of R100 to every South African who earns below a certain minimum income would be around R24 billion per annum. This cost is based on the assumption that existing provisions remain and that individuals already benefiting from these grants would not get the basic income grant. There are therefore extensive budgetary implications for extending social assistance provisions widely enough to ensure that the needs of children infected and affected by HIV/AIDS are met.

Increased expenditure on social assistance could have implications for social development services. The welfare budget is shared between social security (90 per cent), and social development (welfare) services and administration (ten per cent). Approximately seven per cent of the Welfare budget is therefore available for social welfare programmes and services. The White paper for social welfare outlines a shift in emphasis in terms of spending away from cash handouts (social assistance) towards developmental social welfare that fosters independence (Department of Welfare and Population Development, 1997). The target is to move away from the 90/10 breakdown for social security and services respectively, towards an 80/20 breakdown. The increased demand for social security as a result of HIV/AIDS will have an impact on the implementation of this decision and on the delivery of social development services.

Social development services for children include a range of statutory and non-statutory protection, monitoring, intervention and family re-unification services. These services have traditionally focused on identifying and protecting children who are at risk, or intervening in families where abuse or neglect has taken place. The needs of children infected/affected by HIV/AIDS will consume much of the time and energy of social workers, changing the nature of their work and diverting much needed resources away from the issues of child abuse and neglect.

Included in the category of social development services are government subsidised residential care facilities (children's homes). South Africa has approximately 29 000 children in children's homes around the country. Children found in need of care by a children's court are placed in a children's home for a period that should not exceed two years, until suitable long-term care can be found within the child's family or the community. As a result of HIV/AIDS, the nature of care within children's homes is likely to change. Children may spend longer periods within children's homes as it becomes increasingly difficult to find families to care for them. Children's homes will also have to deal with a large number of children in their care who may be HIV-positive. These children may require special medical care, they may have specific dietary requirements and they may be too weak to attend school with their peers. There is a global reluctance to build more orphanages or children's homes to care for the large number of children infected/affected by HIV/AIDS, and an emphasis on initiating and supporting community-based models of care. While this is certainly the preferred option, the increased demand on existing children's homes may well impact on the quality of care offered at these facilities.

**Case Study**

*Why the foster grant needs to be re-thought in light of the switch away from residential to community care and growing numbers of orphans and vulnerable children*

Jardim's House (in Barberton) caters for abused, abandoned and neglected children some of whom are HIV-positive. They have all been placed in the home with a court order. However, the house does not meet the requirements set out by the Department of Health for residential settings, and the Department of Social Development is no longer registering new children's homes. The irony of this is that even though Jardim's House cannot be registered, the social workers from the regional welfare office and the local child welfare society are recommending Sophie Jardim as a foster mother to the Commissioner, who in turn is committing the children to her care. But she is not able to access financial support from the state for all the children in her care . . . There are 14 children living at Jardim's house. Of these eight are receiving some form of state-subsidy – seven foster care grants, and one place-of-safety grant. In order to get around the regulation of

> a maximum of six children per foster care home, some of these children are formally placed with the neighbour but are actually living with Sophie. Three children were placed in the home as a place-of-safety when they were abandoned as babies two years ago. Birth certificates were applied for at the time and have still not been received. As birth certificates are a requirement for a foster care grant, they cannot receive this grant. Neither are they able to receive a place-of-safety grant because the maximum duration for this grant is 12 weeks.'
> (Loening-Voysey and Wilson, 2001)

## References

Adams, J. 2001. 'A Review of Provincial Social Development Budgets 2001'. Institute for Democracy in South Africa. *Budget Brief* 68. Cape Town: Budget Information Service

Barrett, C., N. McKerrow and A. Strode. 1999. 'Consultative Paper on Children Living with HIV/AIDS'. Paper prepared for the South African Law Commission, Pretoria. January.

Cassim, S., H. Perry, M. Sedan and J. Streak. 2000. *Are Poor Children Being Put First: Child Poverty and the Budget 2000*. Cape Town: Institute for Democracy in South Africa.

Child Health Policy Institute and Black Sash. 2000. 'Issue Paper on Social Security for Children in South Africa'. Paper prepared for the Commission of Enquiry into a Comprehensive Social Security System in South Africa. University of Cape Town, Cape Town.

Congress of South African Trade Unions. 2000. *Submission on Establishing a Comprehensive Social Security System for South Africa*. Submitted to the Governmental Committee of Inquiry into Social Security, December 7.

Cullinan, K. 2001. 'Nevirapine is Finally Registered'. HealthE Online News Service, 11 April (accessed March 2002).

Departments of Education, Health and Social Development. 2000. *National Integrated Plan for Children Infected and Affected by HIV/AIDS*. Pretoria.

Department of Health. 1998. *Demographic and Health Survey*. Pretoria.

Department of Health. 2000. *HIV/AIDS/STD Strategic Plan for South Africa 2000–2005*. Pretoria.

Department of Health. 2001. *National HIV & Syphilis Sero-Prevalence Survey of Women Attending Public Antenatal Clinics in South Africa in 2000*. Pretoria.

Department of Social Development. 1999. *A Draft Strategic Framework for Children Infected and Affected by HIV/AIDS*. Pretoria.

Department of Treasury. 2001a. *Budget Review 2001*. Pretoria.

Department of Treasury. 2001b. *National Estimates of Expenditure 2001*. Pretoria.

Department of Welfare and Population Development. 1997. *White Paper for Social Welfare*. Pretoria.

Desmond, C. and J. Gow. 2001. *The Cost Effectiveness of Six Models of Care for Orphan and Vulnerable Children in South Africa*. Pretoria: UNICEF.

Giese, S. 2001. *Social Assistance for Children Made Vulnerable by HIV/AIDS: Submission to the Committee of Inquiry into a Comprehensive Social Security System*. Cape Town: Children's Institute and Child Health Unit, University of Cape Town.

Haarmann, C. 2001. *Social Assistance in South Africa: Its Potential Impact on Poverty*. PhD thesis, University of the Western Cape, Cape Town.

Haarmann, D. 1999. 'The Living Conditions of South Africa's Children'. Applied Fiscal Research Centre, Research Monograph Series, Number 9. University of Cape Town, Cape Town.

Hickey, A. and P. Whelan. 2001. 'HIV/AIDS and Budget 2001'. *Budget Brief* 62. Institute for Democracy in South Africa. Cape Town: Budget Information Service.

Loening-Voysey, H. and T. Wilson. 2001. *Approaches to Caring for Children Orphaned by AIDS and Other Vulnerable Children: Essential Elements for a Quality Service*. Pretoria: UNICEF.

Lyons, M. 2001. 'The Impact of HIV and AIDS on Children, Families and Communities: Risks and Realities of Childhood During the HIV Epidemic'. HIV and Development Program, United Nations Development Program, Issues Paper no. 30. (accessed March 2002).
http://www.undp.org/hiv/publicaitons/issues/english/issue30e.html

May, J., D. Budlender, R. Mokate, C. Rogerson, A. Stavrou and N. Wilkins. 1998. *Poverty and Inequality: Report Prepared for the Office of the Executive Deputy President and the Inter-Ministerial Committee for Poverty and Inequality*. Durban: Praxis Publishing.

Provincial Budget Statements/Estimates of Expenditure. 2001. 2000/01–2003/04 and Budget Speeches.

Russell, M. and H. Schneider. 2000. 'Models of Community-Based HIV/AIDS Care and Support'. In *South African Health Review 2000*, A. Ntuli, N. Crisp, E. Clarke and P. Barron (eds). Durban: Health Systems Trust.

South African National Council for Child Welfare. 1999. *HIV/AIDS and The Care of Children*. Johannesburg.

Smart, R. 1999. *Children Living with HIV/AIDS in South Africa: A Rapid Appraisal*. Johannesburg: Save the Children.

Simelelo, N. 2001. Director, Chief Directorate HIV/AIDS and STDS, National Department of Health. Presentation to the Health Portfolio Parliamentary Committee, 2–5 April.

Steinberg, M., A. Kinghorn, N. Soderlund, G. Schierhout and S. Conway. 2000. 'HIV/AIDS: Facts, Figures and the Future'. In *South African Health Review 2000*, A. Ntuli, N. Crisp, E. Clarke and P. Barron (eds). Durban: Health Systems Trust.

Thorn, A. 2001. 'Children Go Hungry as Grants Fail to Materialise'. HealthE Online News Service, 11 April (accessed March 2002).

CHAPTER 8

# Treatment of HIV/AIDS and Related Illnesses

*Neil McKerrow*

## Introduction
Ideally the holistic management of HIV-infected individuals encompasses a spectrum of interventions aimed at mitigating the impact of the epidemic on the individual and the society in which s/he lives. The full management spectrum comprises prevention, care and support activities that must be broad enough to ensure that the needs of the individual and their family are addressed whilst simultaneously promoting sustainable development of the community in the face of the destructive sequelae of the HIV/AIDS epidemic.

The effective integration of these three elements not only results in reciprocal reinforcement of one another but also serves to establish a sustainable cycle of benefits. For maximal efficacy care and support activities should (Girma and Schietinger, 2000):

- mitigate the impact of the epidemic on the individual, the family and the community;
- enhance the effectiveness of prevention programmes and thereby prevent further HIV transmission;
- promote access to basic health and welfare.

In the case of children, whether infected or affected, this management must occur within and address the context in which the child lives. Interventions addressing the needs of children in the HIV/AIDS epidemic should therefore include the following two components:

- a continuum of prevention, care and support activities;
- a focus on the child, his/her mother and household members, including any alternative caretakers.

It is impossible to divorce the management of children from that of their mothers for the following reasons:

- Preventing HIV infection of women precludes possible vertical transmission of infection to their children.
- Appropriate care of pregnant HIV-positive women reduces the likelihood of vertical transmission of the virus to their children.
- Mothers are generally the primary caretakers of their children and the care of HIV-infected children therefore rests primarily with their mothers.
- Effective care of infected women reduces their morbidity and improves their ability to care for their children irrespective of whether these are infected or not.

In reviewing the treatment of childhood HIV/AIDS it is therefore imperative that some attention is given to the care of HIV-positive women, particularly those who are pregnant.

## *The global response*

During the first twenty years of the epidemic numerous individuals, corporations and national and global bodies have published guidelines, formulated best practice models or recommended responses in one or more areas of HIV/AIDS prevention, care or support. However, given the incurable nature of the infection and the high cost of treatment the responses of developed and developing nations have differed. Developed countries have been able to implement comprehensive preventive, care and support programmes. In contrast, most donor agencies and developing country governments have invested their resources in prevention rather than care and support activities.

The discrepancy in epidemic profiles, available resources and the purpose of HIV/AIDS interventions between the developed and developing world brings into question the relevance of first world guidelines for a third world setting. Most of these guidelines and recommendations represent best practice or optimal responses within the cultural context of the developed world. Their scientific content has global relevance irrespective of cultural and socio-economic variations and as such represent an ideal toward which all govern-ments should aspire. It is therefore important that in formulating their own response programmes the developing world recognise the content of these guidelines. However interventions must be adapted to comply with the cultural and socio-economic circumstances of the countries and communities in which they will be implemented. Numerous guidelines have been developed. The various guidelines cover a wide and comprehensive range of HIV/AIDS-related conditions. These include the care of children, infant feeding practices, tuberculosis (TB), nutritional support, the care of pregnant HIV-positive women and the prevention of mother to child transmission (MTCT).

## *The South African response*

The first co-ordinated South African response to the HIV/AIDS epidemic was produced by the National AIDS Convention of South Africa (NACOSA) in 1994. The NACOSA National AIDS Implementation Plan of 1994 proposed an integrated response of ten strategies fulfilling three objectives.

The implementation plan proposed a holistic response that recognised the rights of all individuals in an affected society – the infected, affected and unaffected – whilst supporting strategies that promote the development of infrastructure, services and a healthy socio-economic environment. The plan also drew specific attention to the status of women and the need for the response to be integrated both horizontally between and vertically within sectors.

Twenty-five specific interventions encompassing 107 activity areas were proposed. By 1994 specific actions within each activity area had been identified and for each action outcomes, responsible parties, timeframes and budgets were described.

Three proposed interventions were of relevance to the treatment of infected children and their mothers:

- Number 3 – improved sexually transmitted disease (STD) control.
- Number 7 – provide information and counselling about HIV, perinatal transmission and related services.
- Number 10 – provide comprehensive healthcare and counselling for people living with HIV/AIDS and their families.

The annual budget for the proposed NACOSA plan was estimated to be R260 million. As this figure exceeded the budget of the HIV/AIDS and STD Programme and many of the structures needed for implementation of the plan did not exist the plan was never adopted by the Department of Health. Instead the National AIDS Programme used the NACOSA plan as the basis for the development of its own strategic plan in 1995/96 (Department of Health, 1994). This plan adopted five key strategies:

- life skills programme targeted at youth;
- the use of mass communication to popularise key prevention concepts in AIDS;

- appropriate treatment and management of patients seeking treatment for STDs;
- increased access to barrier methods;
- the promotion of appropriate care and support.

Four of these five strategies focused on prevention, one addressed management of STDs but none targeted perinatal transmission or the prevention of the vertical infection of children from their mothers.

The provision of appropriate care and support was to be achieved by pursuing nine objectives:

Care:
- develop management protocols for men, women and children;
- improve TB control;
- develop guidelines for appropriate levels of care along a continuum from home to hospital and hospice;
- ensure supply of drugs for treatable opportunistic infections;
- train healthcare workers to provide appropriate care.

Support:
- access counselling and testing through the establishment of at least one AIDS Centre per health district or region;
- improve existing care by increasing the capacity of existing AIDS Centres;
- produce a manual on the content and methodology of a counselling curriculum;
- finance pilot programmes exploring alternative models of counselling.

All of these objectives were relevant in attaining appropriate treatment of children. It is interesting to note that the activities proposed in the development of management protocols for men, women and children were broad and neither advocated nor precluded the use of anti-retroviral (ARV) drugs.

Steps for the implementation of the strategic plan were supported by a detailed business plan outlining specific actions, responsible parties, timeframes and budgets. The estimated budget for the plan was R110 million. Sufficient funds were not available and many of the proposed activities remain unrealised.

The principles adopted in the development of this first strategic plan remain relevant today and were reaffirmed in the development of the HIVSP (Department of Health, 2000a). The latest plan identifies four priority areas and fifteen goals.

The current strategic plan builds on and is more comprehensive than earlier plans. Details of specific goals relevant to treatment issues reveal:

- Support for the syndromic management for STDs by all healthcare practitioners – public, private and traditional.
- The promotion of appropriate family planning amongst HIV-positive women as well as access to voluntary testing and counselling (VTC) in all antenatal services.
- Support for the implementation of clinical guidelines to reduce MTCT during childbirth and labour. Once again strategies are broad and details regarding the use of ARV drugs are absent;
- Recognition of the need to develop treatment guidelines for HIV-positive individuals and to ensure an uninterrupted supply of appropriate drugs. Specific mention is made of drugs for the treatment of TB and other opportunistic infections but not of ARV drugs.
- Support for the strengthening of links between community-based care and institutional care.
- Support for the development of appropriate packages of care within the private sector.

Lead agencies responsible for pursuing each of the above goals are identified in the plan. For all of the activities highlighted above the primary lead agency is the Department of Health at both national and provincial level.

The responses to the HIV/AIDS epidemic outlined in the current strategic plan reflect government policy and not necessarily existing practice. The reality found in many communities and healthcare facilities throughout the country shows excellent plans but in many instances inadequate or incomplete delivery.

**Management of sexually transmitted diseases**

Protocols for the syndromic management of STDs were first developed together with a training manual in 1995 (KwaZulu-Natal Department of Health, 1995). Since then they have been expanded (KwaZulu-Natal Department of Health, 1996a) and updated (Department of Health, 1997). Similar but more comprehensive protocols are included in the Essential Drugs Programme for the primary healthcare level (Department of Health, 1998).

These protocols are both comprehensive and holistic addressing counselling, education and treatment issues relevant to both the public and private sector. Widespread dissemination of the protocols has been achieved to medical practitioners in both the public and private sectors and registered nurses in the public sector. In the public health sector the protocols have been introduced at the primary healthcare level through training courses conducted amongst registered nurses working at that level.

There is no record of whether the protocols are actually used in the private sector whilst in the public sector their use is frequently undermined by interrupted access to the relevant drugs and the need for the ongoing monitoring and training of staff.

In terms of the objectives of the national strategic plan relevant to the control of STDs the current status appears to be as follows:

- Protocols have been developed for the syndromic management of STDs.
- Programmes for the training of healthcare personnel in the use of these protocols have been developed and training workshops have been conducted in many areas of the public sector.
- The extent of application of the protocols within both the public and private sectors needs to be determined.
- The status of collaboration efforts with traditional healers in promoting appropriate health seeking behaviour for STD treatment needs to be established.

**Care of HIV-infected women**

The treatment of HIV-positive women is haphazard, dependent on the enthusiasm, skills and insights of individual healthcare workers in both the public and private sectors. There is little evidence of a widespread, co-ordinated strategy for the treatment of HIV associated illnesses at any level within the public health services.

Since the mid-1990s numerous guidelines for the treatment of HIV-infected adults have been developed locally. Some of these have been produced by individuals acting in their private capacity and do not necessarily reflect official policy or practice (Evian, 1993). Others reflect attempts by some provincial health departments to provide management guidelines for staff in hospitals or primary healthcare facilities (KwaZulu-Natal Department of Health, 1996b). More recently national guidelines have been developed to standardise treatment protocols and provide guidance for those provinces that do not have the capacity to develop their own guidelines (Department of Health, 2000b).

These various guidelines promote reasonably similar approaches to most aspects of HIV care and the quality of the most recent guidelines, the national guidelines, is good. These guidelines form part of a package of nine guidelines that together provide a comprehensive and holistic approach to HIV care in Southern Africa.

Unfortunately distribution and subsequent use of the guidelines has produced yet another comedy of errors in this country's response the epidemic. Ninety thousand copies were produced and made available, on request, to interested parties as part of the HIV/AIDS and STD Directorate's 'Beyond

Awareness' campaign. In KwaZulu-Natal the provincial AIDS Unit received limited numbers of the guidelines, too few for general distribution, and very few health facilities have received copies of the guidelines.

It is well recognised that the production of guidelines is no guarantee that they will be implemented. For this to occur training in their use is required as well as ongoing support and access to the materials prescribed in the guidelines. In 1996, following the development of provincial guidelines, the KwaZulu-Natal HIV/AIDS Clinical Advisory Group conducted a series of workshops in each health region to distribute the guidelines and instruct health staff on their use. Since then, despite a high HIV seroprevalence in the province and a high turnover of staff, no further distribution of guidelines or training workshops for staff has occurred. Use of the guidelines remains extremely limited as very few health workers have a copy, no training has been conducted in their use over the past five years and an erratic supply of essential drugs precludes use of many of the recommendations in the guidelines.

One major deficiency in the guidelines is their failure to provide any information regarding the use of ARV drugs. The rationale behind this failure is the belief that these drugs are too expensive, their use too complicated and the tests required for monitoring their use, viral loads and CD4 counts, not widely available. This deficit has been addressed to some extent by the development of guidelines for ARV therapy in adults by the Southern African HIV Clinicians Society (2000a). The society has recognised that given the constraints of the South African context treatment cannot always be optimal and the guidelines propose acceptable therapeutic alternatives that are currently more affordable and realistic. At present there is limited use of ARV drugs in the public sectors and access is restricted to those patients who are able to purchase the drugs themselves or are fortunate enough to be enrolled in clinical trials.

As part of the comprehensive care package for HIV-positive people the national guidelines produced by the Directorate HIV/AIDS and STD include one on tuberculosis and HIV/AIDS (Department of Health, 2000b). This is an excellent comprehensive guideline outlining the DOTS (Directly Observed Treatment, Short-Course) strategy, the diagnosis and treatment of all forms of TB as seen in HIV-positive adults and children, as well as covering prevention and continuity of care issues.

The 1998 national review of TB control programmes identified many deficiencies in programme delivery. Implementation of these latest guidelines has followed a similar pattern to that experienced with the adult HIV treatment guidelines and without complimentary training and support programmes are unlikely to improve the status of TB control.

With respect to the objectives of the national strategic plan relevant to the care of HIV-positive women the current status appears to be:

- Local guidelines on the management of HIV-infected adults as well as on the uses of ARV drugs have been developed.
- These guidelines are however not widely available.
- Training programmes on the use of these guidelines do not appear to exist.
- Access to an uninterrupted supply of appropriate drugs in the public health service is not guaranteed.
- The medical insurance industry has started to review benefits and coverage for HIV-positive members.
- Policies and programmes have been developed to address the relationship between HIV and TB.
- Implementation of the programme is problematic.

**Programme for the prevention of mother to child transmission of HIV**
The need to introduce a mother-to-child-transmission prevention (MTCTP) programme was first recognised in 1998 when a proposed programme was costed on behalf of the Department of Health (HIV Management Services (Pty) Ltd. 1998). The total cost for introducing this programme – including supplementary staff, staff training, test kits, drugs at a discounted price and milk formula – in all antenatal clinics in the public sector throughout the country was R80 million. The department considered this figure excessive and the proposal was not pursued.

Government decided in 2001 to provide anti-retrovirals to HIV-positive pregnant women. This involves expanding the research sites on Nevirapine treatment with regard to mother to child transmission of HIV/AIDS. The promising results of the HIVNET 012 Nevirapine study in Uganda (Guay et al., 1999) together with further offers of a free supply of drugs have added to public pressure for the introduction of a widespread MTCTP programme. Such a programme was to be introduced in a limited number of sites throughout the country in the first half of 2001. The HIVNET 012 Nevirapine regimen will initially be implemented at two facilities per province, where large numbers of deliveries take place (Department of Treasury, 2001). The Treatment Action Campaign (TAC) has pointed out that the impact of the programme will initially not be that great because the 18 sites only reach about ten per cent of all women attending public antenatal clinics.

Despite a reluctance to provide ARV drugs to pregnant women for the prevention of MTCT, guidelines have been produced outlining other options available to assist healthcare workers and pregnant women in reducing the risk of transmission of HIV from mother to child (Department of Health, 2000c). It is important to recognise that ARV regimens form one element of a total package of care for pregnant women and should not be provided in isolation. However, whilst this guideline provides reasonable insight into all elements of a holistic package and covers behavioural, therapeutic and obstetric interventions as well as advice on infant feeding practices the absence of any discussion on the various ARV regimens currently recommended seriously undermines its value. The infant feeding options available to HIV-positive women are further explored in yet another national guideline (Department of Health, 2000d). This guideline together with all nine national guidelines has not been widely distributed nor supported by staff training workshops.

Plans for the implementation of a national MTCTP programme are at an advanced stage. The programme incorporates voluntary counselling and testing to identify HIV-positive women, antenatal interventions, modified midwifery and infant feeding practices and treatment with Nevirapine. An HIV test is a pre-requisite for access to Nevirapine and ongoing medical support of the HIV-positive woman and her infant including free milk substitutes for six months, vitamin supplements and prophylaxis for opportunistic infections. A major deficiency in the programme is the lack of adequate ongoing psycho-social support for the HIV-positive woman although it is hoped that the programme will act as a catalyst for the development of suitable community-based psycho-social support services and partnerships between the public health services and the community.

With respect to the objectives of the national strategic plan relevant to the prevention of MTCT the current status appears to be the most promising of all aspects of HIV treatment. It is as follows:

- A comprehensive intervention has been developed.
- Planning for the implementation of the intervention is in an advanced stage.
- Unfortunately the intervention is limited to a few pilot sites only and so far no rollout strategy has been developed.

**Care of HIV-infected children**
The response to meeting the needs of HIV-positive children has been similar to that experienced by adults and little evidence of a coordinated treatment strategy exists.

Provincial (KwaZulu-Natal Department of Health, 1996b) and national (Department of Health, 2000e) guidelines for the management of HIV-positive infants and children have been developed. In some instances the production of these guidelines has been supported by one-off training workshops for healthcare workers. However no sustained programmes seem to exist for the ongoing distribution of guidelines or training of healthcare workers.

Whilst the national guidelines are comprehensive, holistic and user friendly they, like the adult guidelines, do not include information on the role of ARV therapy. Once again the HIV clinicians society has filled this gap by publishing its own recommendations (Southern African HIV Clinicians Society, 2000b).

The essential drugs list for paediatric illnesses has no recommendations on HIV treatment but does include one section on occupationally acquired HIV exposure (Department of Health, 1998). Apart from ARV and more specialised drugs all the basic medicines required for the treatment of HIV-associated illnesses in children are included in the list.

The Directorate of Maternal, Child and Women's Health in the KwaZulu-Natal Department of Health has developed a component on the treatment of HIV and associated illnesses for the Integrated Management of Childhood Illnesses (IMCI) programme. This component is being piloted in the Empangeni Health Region. Whilst initial reports suggest that the algorithms are effective they also reveal reluctance amongst IMCI trained staff to utilise them. Further research will be required to identify the reasons for this reluctance, to explore whether these barriers extend to other HIV-related protocols and to identify the steps needed to overcome this reluctance.

The care of HIV-positive children in the private sector is linked to that of their parents and is dependent on the medical insurance scheme to which they subscribe. The benefits available to children are similar to those for adults and as mentioned above an estimated five per cent of HIV-positive patients in the private sector being funded for ARV therapy are children.

No objectives exist in the national strategic plan relating specifically to the treatment of HIV-positive children however children are included as recipients of care and treatment strategies. The current status of child-targeted responses is similar to that outlined above with respect to HIV-positive women:

- Local guidelines on the management of HIV-infected children as well as on the uses of ARV drugs have been developed.
- These guidelines are however not widely available.
- Training programmes on the use of these guidelines do not appear to exist.
- Support services and structures for the successful implementation of the guidelines are also inadequate.

## *Further actions needed to increase the effectiveness of the interventions*

There is no doubt that a wide range of comprehensive and effective strategies have been designed to meet the treatment needs of HIV/AIDS and related illnesses. Unfortunately there is also no doubt that none of these interventions has been successfully implemented on a wide scale anywhere in the country.

In looking at strategies to move from planning to implementation a number of issues need to be reviewed. These include:

- **Partnerships** – in view of the limited resources – financial, material and skills – within the country, especially within the public sector, collaboration with local, national and international parties will be required to supplement these. Possible partners include foreign governments, multi-national agencies, academic institutions and pharmaceutical companies. At present, policies and mechanisms exist for collaboration and the development of partnerships but these are to a large extent limited to the national and to a lesser extent, provincial level.

    Collaboration also occurs through academic institutions. Mechanisms need to be developed to extend the development of partnerships more broadly.

- **Programmes and Communication** – the development of programmes is currently limited to a few role-players who are invariably centrally located within the national Department of Health and academic centres. Neither of these parties are implementing agents. These programmes are then imposed vertically on implementing agents who were never consulted and were not party to their development. Not surprisingly there is little sense of ownership of the programmes and often only half-hearted implementation.

    A current example of this is the Fluconazole programme that is to be implemented for the treatment and secondary prevention of cryptococcal meningitis and oesophageal candidiasis as a joint effort of Pfizer and the national Department of Health.

    Negotiations between Pfizer and a Ministerial Task Team for a two year unlimited donation of Fluconazole from Pfizer to the Department of Health for the above programme were concluded towards the end of 2000. Representation on the ministerial task team was limited with no provincial representatives, no clinicians from the public sector and no paediatricians. The only clinical input was from Pfizer and the South African HIV Clinicians Society. The agreed upon programme is not acceptable to many clinicians working in public sector hospitals due to inadequate diagnostic criteria, contradictory treatment protocols and the exclusion of children.

- **Barriers to the Use of Protocols** – In planning treatment interventions many excellent protocols have been developed. Unfortunately many barriers to the effective use of these protocols appear to exist.

    The development of these protocols is often protracted. Once developed distribution has invariably been inadequate. Ongoing support such as training workshops, easy access to the recommended treatments and ongoing review and updating is lacking. The attitude of many healthcare workers to HIV, and their reluctance to deal comprehensively with HIV-positive individuals, needs to be addressed.

Uninterrupted access to materials and drugs required in the protocols needs to be guaranteed. This is critical as once the issue of partnerships is resolved it is only a matter of time before ARV drugs will be available within the public health service and effective functioning systems need to be in place before ARV regimens can be implemented.

- **Drug Donations** – Now that the debate around parallel imports and drug patents is being resolved the likelihood of partnerships between the government and global pharmaceutical companies is more realistic. Once this occurs, or failing this through the UNAIDS drug initiatives, access to currently unavailable drugs is likely to occur. Mechanisms therefore need to be established for the development of programmes that are relevant at the coalface. This requires a shift from vertical programmes to partnerships between the provinces and national health and the inclusion of more clinicians in planning teams.

- **The Availability of ARV** – It is generally recognised that it is only a matter of time before these become available through the public health sector. It is therefore essential that a process of developing appropriate, innovative, alternative ARV drug regimens start now. A need exists for the development of regional centres of excellence in HIV treatment and ARV use to act focal points for the expansion of programmes throughout all health regions.

- **Ongoing Training** of all healthcare workers in existing programmes and for the implementation of any new programmes for the treatment of HIV and related illnesses is probably the single most important factor following development of appropriate protocols and availability of resources.

It is important to recognise that despite the problems outlined above there are sufficient dedicated and committed personnel in the health sector for the effective implementation of existing treatment protocols. For effective service delivery to become a reality these individuals require effective support. This includes political and administrative commitment to addressing the issues, access to the necessary resources and appropriate skills.

## References

Child Health Unit. 1998. *HIV/AIDS and the Family: A Clinical Guide*. Cape Town: University of Cape Town.
Department of Health. 1994. *Strategy, Business and Structure Plans, 1995–1996*. HIV/AIDS and STD Programme, Pretoria.
Department of Health. 1997. *Protocols for the Management of a Person with a Sexually Transmitted Disease According to the Essential Drugs List*. Directorate HIV/AIDS and STD, Pretoria.
Department of Health. 1998. *Essential Drugs Programme. Standard Treatment Guidelines and Essential Drugs List: Hospital Level, Paediatrics*. Pretoria.
Department of Health. 2000a. *HIV/AIDS & STD Strategic Plan for South Africa, 2000–2005*. Pretoria.
Department of Health. 2000b. *HIV/AIDS Policy Guideline: Tuberculosis and HIV/AIDS*. Directorate HIV/AIDS and STD, Pretoria.
Department of Health. 2000c. *HIV/AIDS Policy Guideline: Prevention of Mother-to-Child HIV Transmission and Management of HIV Positive Pregnant Women*. Directorate HIV/AIDS and STD, Pretoria.
Department of Health. 2000d. *HIV/AIDS Policy Guideline: Feeding of Infants of HIV Positive Mothers*. Directorate HIV/AIDS and STD, Pretoria.
Department of Health. 2000e. *HIV/AIDS Policy Guideline: Managing HIV in Children*. Directorate HIV/AIDS and STD, Pretoria.
Department of Treasury. 2001. *Budget Review 2001*. Pretoria.
Donahue, J. 1998. 'Community-Based Economic Support for Households Affected by HIV/AIDS'. Discussion Paper on HIV/AIDS Care and Support Number 6. Health Technical Services (HTS) Project, Arlington.
Evian, C. 1993. *Primary AIDS Care*. Houghton: Jacana Education.
Girma, M. and H. Schietinger. 2000. 'Integrating HIV/AIDS Prevention, Care, and Support: A Rationale'. Discussion Papers on HIV/AIDS Care and Support. The Synergy Project, United States Agency for International Development, Washington. June.
Guay, L., P. Musoke, T. Fleming, et al. 1999. 'Intrapartum and Neonatal Single-Dose Nevirapine Compared with Zidovudine for Prevention of Mother-to-Child Transmission of HIV-1 in Kampala, Uganda: HIVNET 012 randomised trial'. *Lancet* 354: 795–802.
Harries, A. and D. Maher. 1996. *TB/HIV: A Clinical Manual*. Geneva: World Health Organisation.
HIV Management Services (Pty) Ltd. 1998. *Technical Report: Projections of Costs of Anti-Retroviral Interventions to Reduce Mother-To-Child Transmission of HIV in the South African Public Sector*. Pretoria.
Hunter, S. and J. Williamson. 1998. 'Responding to the Needs of Children Orphaned by HIV/AIDS'. Discussion Paper on HIV/AIDS Care and Support Number 7. Health Technical Services (HTS) Project, Arlington.
Kaplan, J., D. Hu, et al. 1998. 'Preventing Opportunistic Infections in Human Immunodeficiency Virus-Infected Persons: Implications for the Developing World'. Discussion Paper on HIV/AIDS Care and Support Number 4. Health Technical Services (HTS) Project, Arlington.

KwaZulu-Natal Department of Health. 1995. *Syndromic Management of Sexually Transmitted Disease*. Durban.
KwaZulu-Natal Department of Health. 1996a. *Syndromic Management of Sexually Transmitted Disease*. Durban.
KwaZulu-Natal Department of Health. 1996b. *Clinical Guidelines for Children with HIV Infection at Hospitals*. HIV/AIDS Clinical Advisory Group, Durban.
Lambert, J., S. Nogueira and E. Anderson. 1998. *Manual for the Clinical Care of HIV-Infected Pregnant Women*. Santa Monica: Elizabeth Glaser Paediatric AIDS Foundation.
Lazzarini, Z. 1998. 'Human Rights and HIV/AIDS'. Discussion Paper on HIV/AIDS Care and Support Number 2. Health Technical Services (HTS) Project, Arlington.
National AIDS Convention of South Africa. 1994. *Draft National AIDS Implementation Plan*. March. Johannesburg.
Piwoz, E. and E. Preble. 2000. *HIV/AIDS and Nutrition: A Review of the Literature and Recommendations for Nutritional Care and Support in Sub-Saharan Africa*. Washington: Academy for Educational Development.
Sanei, L. 1998. 'Palliative Care for HIV/AIDS in Less Developed Countries'. Discussion Paper on HIV/AIDS Care and Support Number 3. Health Technical Services (HTS) Project, Arlington.
Schietinger, H. and L. Sanei. 1998. 'Systems for Delivering HIV/AIDS Care and Support'. Discussion Paper on HIV/AIDS Care and Support Number 8. Health Technical Services (HTS) Project, Arlington.
Schietinger, H. 1998. *Psychosocial Support for People Living with HIV/AIDS*. Discussion Paper on HIV/AIDS Care and Support Number 5. Health Technical Services (HTS) Project, Arlington.
Southern African HIV Clinicians Society. 2000a. 'Guidelines for ARV Therapy in Adults'. *Southern African Journal of HIV Medicine* 1: 22–26.
Southern African HIV Clinicians Society. 2000b. 'Guidelines for ARV Therapy in Children'. *Southern African Journal of HIV Medicine* 2: 19–30.
UNAIDS. 1998. *HIV-Related Opportunistic Diseases*. Technical Update. Geneva.
UNAIDS. and World Health Organisation. 1999. *HIV in Pregnancy: A Review*. Geneva.
World Health Organisation. 1993. *Guidelines for the Clinical Management of HIV Infection in Children*. Global Program on AIDS. Geneva.
World Health Organisation. 2000. 'Background Paper Prepared for: Technical Consultation on New Data on the Prevention of Mother to Child Transmission of HIV and their Policy Implications'. Geneva.

CHAPTER 9

# Preventing Transmission of HIV

*Rose Smart*

## Background
South Africa's response to the HIV/AIDS epidemic can be divided into three distinct periods; the pre-democracy decade, the period following the first democratic elections and the present which coincides with the rule of President Mbeki.

## *The apartheid responses (pre-1992)*
As early as 1990/91, ANC leaders in exile were speaking about the HIV/AIDS epidemic, warning that it had the potential to result in untold damage and suffering by the end of the century (Chris Hani, Maputo, 1990).

The first responses by Government to the HIV/AIDS epidemic were generated from an AIDS Unit within the national Department of Health and Population Development and about 15 AIDS Training, Information and Counselling Centres (ATICCs) which were situated within larger local authorities. The ATICCs, funded by the AIDS Unit, evolved along different lines in different parts of the country, but all had the core functions described in their name. They developed additional functions in accordance with the expertise of their staff; functions such as media development, research, outreach projects, etc.

The AIDS Unit is best recalled for producing large quantities of small media materials, some quite effective, some very problematic, such as posters with completely different messages for different population groups.

## *Democratic responses (1993–1998)*
It is generally accepted however that the first meaningful response to AIDS emerged with the birth of the National AIDS Convention of South Africa

(NACOSA). In October 1992, a national conference entitled 'South Africa United Against AIDS' was addressed by Nelson Mandela. That event launched the process of developing, firstly, a national AIDS strategy and, subsequently, an implementation plan. Every significant sector was involved – the scale and pace of the process, and the ability for old apartheid adversaries to work together, set it apart as a unique achievement.

**NACOSA National AIDS Plan (1994–1995) Statement of Principles**
- People with HIV and AIDS shall be involved in all prevention, intervention and care strategies.
- People with HIV and AIDS, their partners, families and friends shall not suffer from any form of discrimination.
- The vulnerable position of women in society shall be addressed to ensure that in all respects they do not suffer discrimination, nor remain unable to take effective measures to prevent infection.
- Confidentiality and informed consent with regard to testing and results shall be adhered to at all times
- Education, counselling and healthcare shall be sensitive to the culture, language and social circumstances of all people at all times.
- The government has a crucial responsibility with regard to the provision of education, care and welfare to all people.
- Full community participation in prevention and care shall be developed and fostered.
- All intervention and care strategies shall be subject to critical evaluation and assessment.
- All sectors of government shall be involved in the fight against AIDS, and HIV/AIDS education, prevention and care shall be viewed in a broad social context.
- A holistic approach to education and care shall be developed and sustained.

**Table 9.1    NACOSA National AIDS Plan (1994–1995).**

The NACOSA Plan consisted of three Objectives, containing ten strategies.

**Objective 1:    Prevent HIV transmission**
- prevent sexual transmission
- prevent transmission though blood
- prevent perinatal transmission
- promote policies and programme which address changes in the socio-economic conditions predisposing to the spread of HIV

**Objective 2:    Reduce the personal and social impact of HIV infection**
- provide counselling, care and social support for persons with HIV/AIDS, their families and the community
- provide social welfare services for persons with HIV/AIDS, their families and the community
- reduce the macro-social and macro-economic consequences of HIV/AIDS

**Objective 3:    Mobilise and unify national, provincial, international and local resources**
- mobilise commitment, support and resources
- strengthen national, provincial and local capacities to respond to HIV/AIDS
- strengthen international efforts in the Southern African region

Other role players were non-governmental organisations (NGOs) who were at the forefront of all the early HIV/AIDS service delivery, being the only legitimate structures at that time. The AIDS Programme of the National Progressive Primary Healthcare Network, funded by USAID, was the most extensive of the programmes, with Community AIDS Workers operating in all provinces.

USAID was the most visible donor, supporting a number of NGOs as well as AIDSCAP, an American agency, whose programme focused on traditional healers and on the establishment of a Resource Centre, based in Johannesburg.

**AIDS and the new South Africa: 1994–1998**
In October 1994, Minister Zuma, as Minister of Health in the new democratic government, accepted the NACOSA Plan as the blueprint for the new government's AIDS Programme.

Late in 1995, led by the newly restructured AIDS Directorate in the

Department of Health, five strategies were identified which, in time, were widely embraced by Government and many NGOs. These were:

- life skills programmes targeted at the youth;
- the use of mass communication to popularise key prevention concepts;
- appropriate treatment and management of clients seeking treatment for sexually transmitted diseases (STDs);
- increased access to barrier methods;
- the promotion of appropriate care and support.

Extensive funding was made available both from government as well as from donors, primarily the European Union, and AIDS was given the status of a Presidential Lead Project (along with 20 other social priorities), which resulted in yet further funding from the Reconstruction and Development Programme. The sudden injection of bilateral funding to Government coincided with the withdrawal of donor funds to NGOs and this period saw the demise of many AIDS Service Organisations, most notably the AIDS Programme of the National Progressive Primary Healthcare Network.

The National HIV/AIDS and STD Programme was operationalised by the National Directorate: HIV/AIDS and STDs, the nine provincial HIV/AIDS and STD structures and the ATICCs (20 at this stage). In addition, a number of NGOs were either funded or sub-contracted to run projects or to provide services.

The Mission Statement of the National HIV/AIDS and STD Programme was: 'To reduce the transmission of STDs (including HIV infection) and provide appropriate treatment, care and support for those infected and affected, through collaborative efforts within all levels of government, using the NACOSA National AIDS Plan as the terms of reference. The Programme is committed to challenging prejudice and discrimination wherever it occurs.'

In mid-1997, a national review of the response to the AIDS epidemic took place to 'Review the Past, Plan the Future, Work Together'. The review findings indicated:

- the need for leadership, and political and public commitment;
- the importance of meaningful involvement of people living with HIV and AIDS;
- the centrality of an inter-departmental and inter-sectoral response;
- the critical capacity building requirements;
- the benefits of close collaboration with the TB Programme;
- the urgency to address human rights abuses and to reduce stigmatisation.

**Table 9.2  Outline of HIV/AIDS/STD Strategic Plan for South Africa (2000–2005) (HIVSP).**

| |
|---|
| **The primary goals are to:**<br>Reduce the number of new HIV infections (especially among youth)<br>Reduce the impact of HIV/AIDS on individuals, families and communities<br><br>Four main areas constitute the Plan:<br><br>**Prevention**<br>Goal 1: Promote safe and healthy sexual behaviour<br>Goal 2: Improve the management and control of STDs<br>Goal 3: Reduce mother to child transmission<br>Goal 4: Address issues relating to blood transfusion and HIV<br>Goal 5: Provide appropriate post-exposure services<br>Goal 6: Improve access to voluntary HIV testing and counselling<br><br>**Treatment, care and support**<br>Goal 7: Provide treatment, care and support services in health facilities<br>Goal 8: Provide adequate treatment, care and support services in the community<br>Goal 9: Develop and expand the provision of care to children and orphans<br><br>**Monitoring, research and surveillance**<br>Goal 10: Ensure AIDS vaccine development<br>Goal 11: Investigate treatment and care options<br>Goal 12: Conduct policy research<br>Goal 13: Conduct regular surveillance<br><br>**Human and legal rights**<br>Goal 14: Create an appropriate social environment<br>Goal 15: Develop an appropriate legal and policy environment |

## *The Mbeki challenge (1998 onwards)*

In October 1998, Deputy President Mbeki, on behalf of President Mandela, addressed the nation and launched the Partnership Against AIDS – the aim being to broaden and formalise the participation by all sectors in the response to the epidemic.

Many sectors responded with pledges to join the partnership, notably people living with HIV/AIDS, women's and youth organisations, the religious sector, labour, organised business, and sport and entertainment.

Early in 2000, an HIV/AIDS/STD Strategic Plan (2000–2005) was developed. It stated that all government departments, organisations and stakeholders will use this document as the basis to develop their own strategic and operational plans so that all our initiatives as a country as a whole can be harmonised to maximise efficiency and effectiveness.

The aim in the National Strategic Plan (2000–2005) is for every government ministry and every sector (parastatal, NGO, private, faith-based, youth and women) to have dedicated HIV/AIDS focal persons. The establishment of structures at district level is recognised in order to ensure implementation of the plan.

A target of R10 per person per year has been set as the resource standard – or a total of R400 million per year for the whole country.

As the third decade of the AIDS epidemic is entered, there is abundant evidence that Government is serious about addressing the epidemic. Media coverage is extensive and progressively more responsible. Efforts to de-stigmatise AIDS and ensure meaningful participation of people living with HIV and AIDS continue and the human rights lobby remains very active.

## *Analysis of current prevention responses*
### Legal, ethical and human rights context

In line with international trends, activists, lawyers, counsellors and people living with HIV and AIDS have consistently rallied for a human rights approach to the epidemic, arguing that the only way to reduce the growth of the epidemic is to encourage every individual to take responsibility for their own health. Thus rather than attempting to protect the uninfected majority by removing the infected minority from society, the answer lies in protecting the rights of those infected.

> The protection and promotion of human rights are necessary both to protect the inherent dignity of persons affected by HIV/AIDS and to achieve the public health goals of reducing vulnerability to HIV infection, lessening the adverse impact of HIV/AIDS on those affected, and empowering individuals and communities to respond to HIV/AIDS. (UNAIDS, 1997)

It has never been attempted to halt the epidemic by introducing a range of repressive laws. Indeed, the constitution and a host of other non-discrimination laws should protect people living with HIV/AIDS. However, the reality is that many HIV-positive people face violations of their rights on a daily basis. For example: healthcare workers obtain consent to test an employee for hepatitis B but then test their blood for HIV without their knowledge; day care centres refuse to take HIV-positive children; and employers refuse to allow HIV-positive people to join the company medical aid schemes.

## Prevention efforts

As a starting point it is necessary to highlight the awareness versus behaviour change dilemma that remains perhaps the most elusive goal for developing countries seeking to appropriately respond to the HIV/AIDS epidemic.

In general, levels of awareness of HIV/AIDS are high (though some myths and misconceptions persist). There is however little evidence of behaviour change. This is indicative of the complex nature of perceived vulnerability and the lack, particularly for young people and other vulnerable groups, of any real self-efficacy related to sexual decision making.

That stated, how effective have the responses been to the prevention challenges? The critique of key prevention activities by government and at community level focuses on the period from 1997 to the present.

Amongst the significant prevention achievements in this period are:

- the life skills programme;
- mass media campaigns;
- the STD programme;
- the condom programme;
- voluntary counselling and testing (VCT).

Each of these programmes is summarised below and reviewed, followed by a description of selected targeted community level prevention interventions that have the potential to become best practice examples. The option to present just a few examples has been selected as it is simply not possible to describe and critique all community-level prevention initiatives.

## Life skills programmes for youth

The SA Schools Act No. 84 of 1996 regulates amongst other things, admissions and expulsions and provides protection for learners who are infected with HIV. The National Education Policy on HIV/AIDS, Government Notice 1926 of 1998 covers the management of HIV/AIDS in schools. It is based on principles of non-discrimination, confidentiality, education, and measures to manage HIV/AIDS within the school environment.

In 1997, 840 Master Trainers and 9 034 secondary school teachers were trained in life skills and HIV/AIDS and quantities of materials were purchased to resource the schools. This programme was managed by the Department of Health – only recently has the Department of Education taken over as the lead Department. In 1999, the life skills programme was extended into selected primary schools, and piloted in ten schools in the Free State and ten in the Northern Province. The roll out of this programme could potentially reach 21 304 primary schools and 8 497 388 primary school learners.

Cabinet, on 24 November 1999, approved funds amounting to R450 million for an integrated response to the epidemic focusing on children and youth. In 2000/01, R75 million was allocated to the integrated strategy – 57 per cent of which was for life skills education.

In support of the life skills programme which primarily targets youth in school, a youth programme (the South African AIDS Youth Programme or SAYP) has been established which targets youth through social mechanisms and youth organisations.

One life skills product that has been successfully and extensively used is Stepping Stones, a workshop series designed to promote sexual and reproductive health. It addresses questions of gender, sexual health, HIV/AIDS, gender violence, communication and relationship skills. In doing so it recognises that sexual relationships are always situated within a broader context of relationships with sexual partners, families and the community or society in which people live. These influences substantially determine how people behave.

The Stepping Stones manual is intended to be used in its entirety with peer group participants who work through all sessions, each building on previous ones. It is designed for use with people of any age and both genders. Originally developed for use in small, rural communities in Uganda, it has now been adapted for use here.

In the area of life skills programmes for the youth, the challenge remains to utilise peer education on a large scale as an effective way to influence adolescent sexual behaviour. Discrete projects, targeting both in-school youth as well as out-of-school youth, offer hopes of success, but these have not been rolled out on any large scale.

### Mass media campaigns
BEYOND AWARENESS

The Beyond Awareness communication campaigns, recognising that the levels of awareness around HIV/AIDS were in fact high, took the debate to a more personal level, encouraging people to confront their vulnerability, and linking them to resources such as the AIDS Helpline operated by Life Line.

Beyond Awareness II was a multimedia communication campaign that was conducted in two phases over a three year period (1998–2000). The objectives of the campaign were to:

- intensify communication of key messages around the HIV/AIDS epidemic directed primarily at youth;
- develop and distribute communications resources that can support action around HIV/AIDS;

- promote social action through targeted projects – specifically these included the AIDS Memorial Quilt Project, a Tertiary Institutions Project and a Media workers Project;
- build capacity amongst HIV/AIDS communicators and strategists through conducting key research;
- conduct appropriate behavioural research in support of HIV/AIDS communication and evaluate various aspects of the campaign.

Key achievements were the following:

- More than 80 different items were developed including multilingual leaflets, posters, resource guides, booklets, stickers, and utility items. These were used in multiple contexts, such as counselling, training, health education promotion, workshops, forums, cultural activities (e.g. dance, drama, music), youth camps, exhibitions, libraries and resource centres, clinic consultations, door-to-door visits, street campaigns, events (e.g. festivals, HIV/AIDS day focuses, orientations, parades), public transport campaigns, and distribution to friends and relatives.
- A central office was established to handle requests for materials. During 1999/2000 over 25 million items were distributed to thousands of organisations including national and provincial government departments, NGOs, community-based organisations (CBOs), and a wide range of sectoral organisations.
- The wearing of the red ribbon was widely promoted. This is a recognisable icon that can be associated with a wide range of HIV/AIDS communication and social action oriented activities. The ribbon allows HIV/AIDS to move from the invisible to the visible, and also allows individuals to personalise their endorsement of HIV/AIDS issues by wearing the ribbon.

THE AIDS HELPLINE

The AIDS helpline is a toll-free national service that was initiated in 1992. It provides an important opportunity for dialogue, whilst at the same time offering accurate basic information, counselling and referral. The line also plays an important role in breaking down myths, and creates the opportunity for a confidential interaction with a trained counsellor. As a result of various Beyond Awareness activities, there was an increase of over 320 per cent in calls to the toll-free AIDS helpline as shown in Figure 9.1.

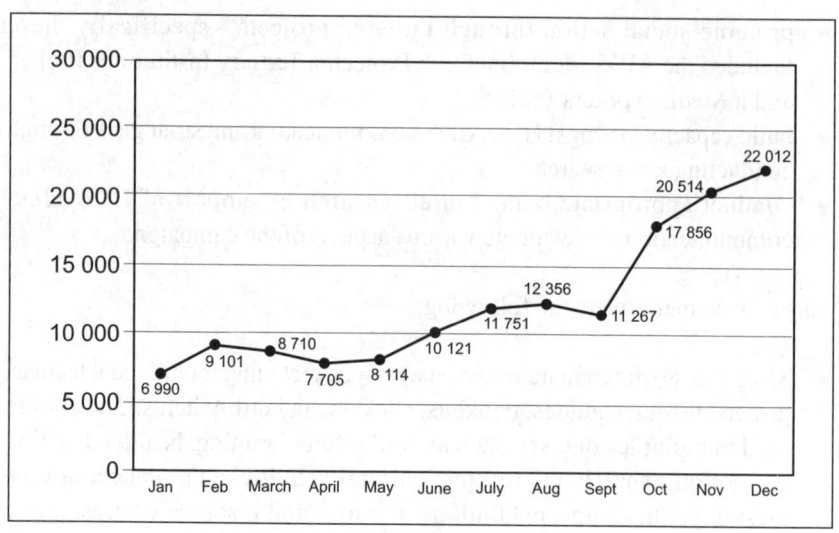

**Figure 9.1 Calls to the AIDS Helpline – 1999.**

SOUL CITY
Soul City is a national multi-media educational/entertainment project that integrates health and development issues into prime time television and radio dramas, backed up by full colour easy to read booklets. For the past few years, HIV/AIDS has been one of the topics covered in each series. The Soul City evaluation released in 2001, shows that the programmes reach more than 16.2 million people, and that personal values are shifting towards greater acceptance, inclusion, support and the normalisation of living with people who are HIV-positive.

Both qualitative and quantitative evidence show that Soul City has played a major role in increasing accurate knowledge about HIV/AIDS, and in shifting people's attitudes, subjective social norms, intermediate practice as well as direct practice towards sustaining safer sexual behaviours.

In the future communication campaigns will need to focus on care – both direct care such as counselling, treatment and care of the ill, as well as the creation of a climate that minimises discrimination and stigmatisation through social mobilisation and advocacy for human rights.

**Syndromic management**
Since 1996/7, STD management protocols based on the syndromic approach have been the gold standard in the public sector. Syndromic STD manage-ment provides high quality STD care by treating people with one or more STDs with the most effective drugs at their first point of contact with the health service.

The emphasis is on rapid treatment and increasing people's access to sexual and reproductive healthcare. The syndromic approach is well-suited to primary healthcare services in resource poor settings because it does not rely upon expensive or inaccessible laboratory tests for diagnosis.

Health workers are trained to diagnose (by taking a history confirmed by examination) and treat on the basis of the identification of a syndrome. A STD syndrome is the grouping of symptoms (given by the patient) and clinical signs shown in the examination by the health worker.

Once the syndrome has been diagnosed, treatment is provided for the majority of organisms known to be responsible for that particular syndrome. The health worker is guided by a flowchart (or algorithm) to the most effective treatment for a given set of signs and symptoms.

Additionally, health workers are trained in other STD management strategies including contact tracing to ensure that their sexual partners are assessed and treated, provision of male and female condoms, counselling and patient education to assist them in taking the full course of treatment.

**Periodic presumptive treatment**
Periodic presumptive treatment (PPT) is sometimes called selective mass treatment. It means that patients are offered regular (periodic) treatment with an antibiotic which is known to be effective against many different STDs. It is presumptive since the patients have not been diagnosed with an STD. On the basis of previous research showing that the majority of the group have curative STDs, it is presumed that they have STDs requiring treatment. Groups usually targeted for PPT are women at high risk who have multiple sexual partners or sex workers.

The use of a new antibiotic such as azithromycin offers the opportunity to cure many different STDs (including gonorrhoea, chlamydia, chancroid and possibly syphilis) with a single oral dose. Previously, similar approaches used injections of drugs like penicillin, which had a major impact on syphilis, but less effect on other STDs because of drug resistance in the other STDs.

The approach offers the opportunity to treat many different STDs with a single dose of antibiotic without an injection. It is expected that such an approach will rapidly reduce the number of infections already present as well as curing new infections acquired after the approach has been started.

An obvious advantage is that it can be implemented rapidly while improvements to clinical STD services are being implemented. The major disadvantage is that many patients will be treated when they do not have infections. For this reason, it is very important to know that STD rates are high before the approach is implemented.

The most significant challenge still to be resolved relates to the treatment of STDs by the private sector, specifically doctors. A 1997 study not only showed that many people with STDs select doctors as their favoured healthcare provider (5 million cases per year), but that the treatment they receive may well be inadequate (Dartnell et al., 1997).

Percentage of doctors whose reported regimens of treatment were judged to be effective:

- 29 per cent for the syndrome of urethral discharge (in men);
- 15 per cent for the syndrome of genital ulcer;
- 6 per cent for the syndrome of vaginal discharge (in women);
- 4 per cent for pelvic inflammatory disease (in women).

## Barrier methods

The Department of Health has prioritised condom distribution through a systematic annual procurement programme, supported by distribution through clinics and other sites (71 per cent of condom users report that they obtain supplies from clinics or community health centres). Access to barrier methods, primarily male condoms, has been greatly improved despite some problems with quality control. In 1999, 150–160 million condoms were distributed free of charge.

National condom week, every year in February, focuses attention on safer sex. The slogan 'Get wise, Condomise' has been used on a wide range of media including radio, print and outdoor.

In addition to free condoms, male condoms are available for purchase from many retail outlets. Subsidised condoms are available through outlets that are part of the social marketing network. Female condoms are available from selected clinics or for sale from some retail outlets.

Despite improved access there are still significant barriers to condom use in certain areas and particularly for many youth. A survey conducted recently by Condom Concepts and Latex Surgical Products highlighted that young adults:

- do not trust free condoms;
- think that they are of inferior quality.

## Voluntary counselling and testing

The Bill of Rights (section 14) provides for the right to privacy and this implies the right to confidentiality regarding medical information – including HIV status. The right to bodily integrity implies that medical treatment (including HIV testing) may only be carried out with the informed consent of the person concerned.

Reviews of studies on the effects of HIV/AIDS counselling on risk behaviour indicate that VCT is an effective secondary prevention strategy for HIV-infected persons and discordant couples. As a primary prevention strategy to limit the spread of infection to those not yet infected there are still opposing points of view.

On-going attempts are being made to improve access to voluntary counselling and testing. Minimum standards of counsellor training have been set as well as guidelines for maintaining quality and for mentoring lay counsellors have been set. Training and deploying lay counsellors in sites where testing is available has been tried with various levels of intensity in most provinces.

An evaluation of counselling, conducted by the University of Natal (Pietermaritzburg) in 2000 showed that:

- Counselling services have mainly been developed around HIV testing. These are situated largely in healthcare settings and remain underdeveloped and under-resourced at community level.
- Counselling services are still not fully operational along a continuum of care from before infection through to illness, death and bereavement counselling.
- Counselling services are vulnerable to inconsistencies in funding and to changes in funding administration and requirements.
- Lay counsellors did not differ from nurse counsellors on any measure of competence or quality of counselling.
- The current cadre of counselling organisations, sites and personnel represent a committed, dedicated and competent solid foundation on which to develop and extend the continuum of counselling, care and support services essential in impacting on the epidemic.

The challenges will be to balance the promotion of counselling with effective and adequate services. The issues of counsellor selection, knowledge and skill, diversity in counselling approaches and capacity in the delivery of counselling services will need to be addressed. In addition there needs to be continuous review of whether services are client-centred or tending rather towards educative and directive sessions.

## *Emerging best practice examples in prevention*
### Mothusimpilo

The Mothusimpilo project, started in January 1998, initially as a research-driven project, has achieved world renown in describing the complexities of an emerging epidemic and testing those interventions that collectively can be an effective response to HIV/AIDS. Mothusimpilo serves a population of

,000 residents and 50 000 migrant mine workers in the Carletonville/ Khutsong area of Gauteng. The area is typical of gold mining towns. Once prosperous, the community has, in the last 15 years, faced multiple retrenchments, and all the socio-economic strains that accompany the downsizing of such a major industry. This downsizing coincided with the arrival of the HIV/AIDS epidemic. Surveys showed that HIV infections were escalating at an alarming rate – a six per cent HIV prevalence in 1995, 15 per cent in 1997 and by 2001, 40 per cent in males, 60 per cent in females, 70 per cent amongst sex workers and 40 per cent amongst mine workers. In response to this, Mothusimpilo was conceived as a multi-pronged strategy to minimise new HIV and STD infections. Its foundations are:

- optimal STD treatment; and
- the promotion of, and support for, safer sex.

INTERVENTIONS TO ENSURE OPTIMAL STD TREATMENT
- Syndromic management for clients with STDs – in public sector health clinics, at mine medical services and by private sector healthcare providers – is the gold standard which is promoted. Traditional healers are encouraged to refer clients for STD treatment to public sector health clinics.
- Periodic presumptive treatment of STDs in women who have multiple sexual partners, is a revolutionary initiative with great potential to prevent new HIV infections.

INTERVENTIONS TO PROMOTE AND SUPPORT SAFER SEX
- Peer education on the mines and at hot spots where commercial sex occurs ensures that the correct messages are widely disseminated.
- Condom promotion and distribution through multiple outlets in the community and workplace means easy access to protection.

Mothusimpilo also supports a number of community-based interventions that have emerged to meet the demands of the maturing epidemic. These are the Youth Friendly Services providing HIV/AIDS and reproductive support to youth in- and out-of school, and the Home-Based Care Services that provide care and support to people living with HIV and AIDS, to community members with terminal conditions and to their families, including children in distress.

**Key achievements in 2001**
- Within a period of 6 months, there has been a 71 per cent reduction in STDs in women at high risk who are receiving PPT.
- This in turn has led to a dramatic 51 per cent reduction in STDs amongst the local mine workers.

- The contact slip for partners of STD clients has been introduced throughout the district, resulting in a dramatic increase in STD health-seeking behaviour.

**The AIDS train**
The 'On the Right Track' AIDS train which is in effect a moving AIDS conference, travelled around the country in 1999 and 2000 featuring discussions on AIDS, and meeting delegates from government, women's organisations, and the media. Phase two planned to highlight issues involving women and AIDS, soliciting information from women about their concerns and recommendations. The aim is to mobilise and organise women from all walks of life to fight AIDS.

**Long distance road freight and cross border initiatives**
A new project aimed at containing HIV/AIDS in the road freight industry was recently launched. 'Trucking Against Aids' is a joint project of the Transport Department, trade unions and the road freight industry (Engen, Mercedes-Benz and the Road Transport Industry Education and Training Board). In another project, cross-border interventions in high transmission areas are presently being implemented along the Durban–Lusaka corridor.

**Other prevention initiatives**
A programme to train traditional healers was successfully implemented in all provinces.

The Metropolitan Group has launched an AIDS information website for Africa, just one of their many attempts to raise awareness and create an environment for effective prevention.

Forums that deal with prevention as one aspect of their role include the Civil Military Alliance Against AIDS and the Inter-Departmental Committee of representatives from national government departments which aims to develop HIV/AIDS workplace policies and minimum HIV/AIDS programmes for all government departments.

**References**
Dartnell, E., H. Schneider, Z. Hlapshwayo and F. Clews. 1977. *STD Management in the Private Sector*. Centre for Health Policy, University of the Witwatersrand, Johannesburg.
Life Line. 1998. *Beyond Awareness Campaign*. Johannesburg.
National AIDS Convention of South Africa. 1994. *Draft National AIDS Implementation Plan*. Johannesburg.

South African Bill of Rights. 1996. Chapter 2 in Constitution of the Republic of South Africa Act 1996.
UNAIDS. 1997. *HIV/AIDS and Human Rights Guidelines*. Geneva.

# CONCLUSION

CHAPTER 10

# Time for the Next Steps

*Jeff Gow and Chris Desmond*

In this book the latest statistics, thoughts and writings on the impacts of the HIV/AIDS epidemic on the children of South Africa as well as a comprehensive discussion of current interventions and their effectiveness to address the situation has been drawn together.

The impacts of the HIV/AIDS epidemic on children are numerous. Children will be infected, become ill and die, others will live to see their parents or other loved ones become increasingly sick and eventually succumb. Still more children will be affected by the impacts on the health, education and welfare system and all children will be affected in one way or another by widespread adult deaths and the broader economic implications of the epidemic. These impacts are violations of the basic rights of children. Many of these children already live in poverty and HIV/AIDS will serve only to make their bad situation worse. The outlook is gloomy, but there are steps which can be, and in some cases already are being, taken to mitigate these impacts.

Participation is essential if responses are to be appropriate and implementable. Children, non-governmental organisations (NGOs), community-based organisations (CBOs) and all levels of government need to be involved in the development, implementation and monitoring of interventions. This book has attempted to highlight the importance of allowing children and those who care for them to exercise their right to be involved in decisions that affect them. Who better to identify priorities than those who experience the impacts? Furthermore many NGOs, CBOs and individuals are already responding to many of the impacts and much can be learnt from their experience, and their involvement in any expansion will be critical for success.

There are many other important and pressing issues relating to HIV/AIDS and children in South Africa. This book has concentrated on the symptomatic impacts and responses to them. Serious consideration needs also to be given to the underlying problems in society, which have lead to these problems and in some ways the impacts. Why are so many adults and children living in poverty? Why are the health, welfare and education systems already so strained? Why has the socio-economic and political environment allowed, and at times promoted, the spread of HIV? Why does macro-economic policy constrain public spending in the midst of a disaster?

In the absence of adequate inter-generational provision for the future of AIDS-affected children, Cohen (2000) observed: 'A generation is thus emerging with poor health status, few skills (not even those necessary for rural development), low levels of literacy and numeracy, little or no access to financial and other real assets (where their property and other rights will often have been infringed), and who has been deprived of the normal processes of socialisation and social inclusion.'

The time for action to reverse these impacts more effectively is now.

(www.unicef-icdc.org)

# AIDS, PUBLIC POLICY AND CHILD WELL-BEING[1]

edited by
Giovanni Andrea Cornia

## Table of contents

Introduction  *Giovanni Andrea Cornia*

### Part I: Overview of the HIV/AIDS Impact and Policy-Programme Proposals

1. Overview of the Impact and Best Practice Policy and Programme Responses in Favour of Children Living a World Affected by HIV/AIDS
   *Giovanni Andrea Cornia*

### Part II. The Social and Economic Impact of HIV/AIDS on Children: Evidence from Eight Country Case Studies

2. The Impact of HIV/AIDS on Children: Lights and Shadows in the 'Successful Case' of Uganda
   *Darlison Kaija and Robert Basaza*

3. The Impact of a Growing HIV/AIDS Epidemic on the Kenyan Children
   *Boniface O. K'Oyugi and Jane Muita*

4. The Socio-Economic Impact of HIV/AIDS on Children in a Low Prevalence Context: The Case of Senegal
   *Cheikh Ibrahima Niang and Paul Quarles van Ufford*

5. HIV/AIDS, Lagging Policy Response and Impact on Children: The Case of Côte d'Ivoire
   *Jacques Pégatiénan and Didier Blibolo*

6. The Current and Future Impact of the HIV/AIDS Epidemic on South Africa's Children
   *Chris Desmond and Jeff Gow*

7. The Perinatal AIDS and Orphan Problem in the Aftermath of Successful Control of the HIV Epidemics: The Case of Thailand
   *Wattana S. Janjaroen and Suwanee Khamman*

8. HIV/AIDS and Children in the Sangli District of Maharashtra (India)
   *Ravi K. Verma, S.K. Singh, R. Prasad and R.B. Upadhyaya*

9. Limiting the Potential Future Impact of HIV/AIDS on Children in Yunnan (China)
   *China HIV/AIDS Socio-Economic Impact Study Team*

**Part III: The Sectoral Impact of HIV/AIDS on Child Wellbeing and Policy Responses**

10. HIV/AIDS and Economy: Impact and Policy Options
    *Giovanni Andrea Cornia and Fabio Zagonari*

11. Poverty and HIV/AIDS: Impact, Coping and Mitigation Policy
    *Tony Barnett and Alan Whiteside*

12. Mitigating the Impact of HIV/AIDS on Education Supply, Demand and Quality
    *Carol Coombe*

13. The Impact of HIV/AIDS on the Health System and Child Health
    *Giovanni Andrea Cornia, Mahesh Patel and Fabio Zagonari*

14. Increasing the Access to Antiretroviral Drugs to Moderate the Impact of AIDS: An Exploration of Alternative Options
    *Pierre Chirac*

15. The Impact of HIV/AIDS on Orphans and Program and Policy Responses
    *Stanley Phiri and Douglas Webb*

**Note**

1. This project was started in 2000 at the UNICEF's Innocenti Research Centre under the leadership of the Director of the Centre and of the Regional Director of the Eastern and Southern Africa Region Office (ESARO) of UNICEF. Giovanni Andrea Cornia

of the University of Florence took care of the framing, implementation and finalisation of the study. The project could not have been implemented without the support of many colleagues in many UNICEF offices around the world. The financial support of the Italian Government and UNICEF ESARO is gratefully acknowledged.

**The papers included in this study present the views of their authors and not those of UNICEF.**